MENTAL HEALTH
NURSING

Mosby's Review Series

MENTAL HEALTH NURSING

Paulette D. Rollant, PhD, MSN, RN, CCRN
President, Multi-Resources, Inc.
Grantville, Georgia

Denise B. Deppoliti, MS, RN, CS
Director of Nursing, Clinical Resource and Development
St. Joseph's Hospital Health Center
Syracuse, New York

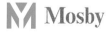

St. Louis Baltimore Boston Carlsbad Chicago Naples New York Philadelphia Portland
London Madrid Mexico City Singapore Sydney Tokyo Toronto Wiesbaden

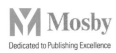

Dedicated to Publishing Excellence

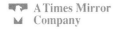

A Times Mirror
Company

Vice-President and Publisher: Nancy L. Coon
Senior Editor: Susan R. Epstein
Associate Developmental Editor: Laurie K. Muench
Project Manager: Carol Sullivan Weis
Designer: Sheilah Barrett
Manufacturing Supervisor: Karen Lewis
Cover Illustrator: Susan Swan

Printed in the United States of America
Composition by Shepherd, Inc.
Printing/binding by R.R. Donnelly

Mosby–Year Book, Inc.
11830 Westline Industrial Drive
St. Louis, MO 63146

International Standard Book Number 0-8151-7247-8

97 98 99 / 9 8 7 6 5 4 3 2

Diane F. Dettmore, RN, BSN, MA, MEd, EdD
Freelance Editor
West Hartford, Connecticut

Carol Flom, RN, BSN, MEd, MS
Nursing Instructor
Minneapolis Community College
Minneapolis, Minnesota

REVIEWERS

To Dan, Mom, Dad, Joanne, Joe, Alan, and Amy
Paulette Rollant

To Bernice Bramley, my sons, Bruce and Brian,
and my deceased father, Amos Bramley
Denise Deppoliti

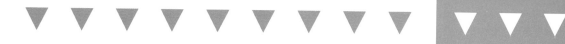

HOW CAN *MOSBY'S REVIEW SERIES* BE USED?

Mosby's Review Series is designed to help you obtain the most from your preparation and study time for your nursing exams. These books should be used to review essential concepts, theory, and content prior to nursing courses, challenge, certification, or licensing examinations. The review series can be used to prepare for clinical experiences and as a quick reference when providing care of clients. Mosby's Review Series consists of five books:

Maternity Nursing
Medical-Surgical Nursing
Mental Health Nursing
Pediatric Nursing
Nursing Pharmacology

The series is designed to highlight important information related to the specific content. It is not meant to provide a comprehensive, in-depth coverage of the selected area of nursing. The reference list at the end of each book is a compilation of resources used to develop these books. These references as well as other texts should be consulted when a more comprehensive discussion of a particular topic is desired. Use these books to jog your memory, to reinforce what you know, to guide you to identify what you don't know, and to lead you to appropriate sources for more details. If you are in a formal education setting, these books are not intended to be considered as a substitute for attending classes or completing required reading assignments.

Used correctly these books can help you:
1. Increase your ability to prioritize in clinical situations while using the nursing process.
2. Increase your ability to remember essential content.
3. Increase your productivity in studying to leave some time for you and your family.
4. Apply new behaviors for improvement of your testing skills.
5. Evaluate your strengths and weakness related to content areas or testing situations.

WHAT IS UNIQUE ABOUT *MOSBY'S REVIEW SERIES?*

1. Computer disks of exams
2. Comprehensive rationales
3. Test-taking tips
4. Chapter format
5. References for further reading

Computer Disk

Each book in the series has a comprehensive exam on computer disk. For your convenience, the exam is also included in the book. The answers for the comprehensive exams, like the end of the chapter questions, include the answers, comprehensive rationales, and test-taking tips.

Comprehensive Rationales

These include answers and rationales for each option in each test question.

Test-Taking Tips

These tips aid in your decision-making and facilitate the development of your logical thinking for the selection of the correct answers, especially if you have narrowed your choice to two options.

Chapter Format

Each chapter contains an easy-to-follow format divided into five sections:

Study Outcomes: provides an advanced organizer approach to what is in each chapter

Key Terms: includes the most common difficult terms to recall

Content Review: is organized and structured by the nursing process to help you identify what is most important

▼ All information within each heading is prioritized
▼ Nursing diagnoses are prioritized
▼ Goals are client-centered
▼ Client teaching content is focused for in-hospital and at-home clinical settings
▼ Home care content is included
▼ Older adult alerts are included where applicable
▼ Evaluation criteria includes decision-making tools concerning which actions to take when client's clinical status shows improvement or deterioration
▼ Many tables, charts, and figures contrast, cluster, and simplify information for ease of remembering

Review Questions: stand-alone, 4-option multiple choice

Answers, Rationales, and Test-Taking Tips:

▼ Comprehensive rationales: given for each option to explain why it is correct or incorrect

▼ Test-taking tips: give strategies to use in situations such as when options are narrowed to two or when you have no idea of a correct answer

References
Current references are suggested for further study if more in-depth discussion is needed.

WHAT'S IN *MOSBY'S REVIEW SERIES: MENTAL HEALTH NURSING?*

Mosby's Review Series: Mental Health Nursing begins with a conceptual framework for the psychiatric nurse. Initially, the mental health-mental disorder continuum is presented. Issues such as legal, ethical, and the nurse's role are included to complete the essential framework related to mental health nursing. Chapter 6 focuses on the therapeutic treatment modalities, including psychotherapy, milieu, activity, group, and somatic therapies. Family interventions are also covered.

The remaining chapters provide essential content for the more common disorders. Initially, the disorders presented are: psychosexual, personality, eating, anxiety, somatoform, and dissociative. Abusive type disorders covered are substance abuse and situations of abusive/self-destructive behaviors. The book concludes with disorders of the affective, psychotic, paranoid, and the developmental related disorders of childhood, adolescence, the older adult, and organic mental disorders.

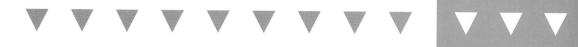

I express my heartfelt gratitude to those who have endured with me throughout this publication opportunity for a nursing review series: an adventure from idea to reality.

I especially want to thank the following people:

Beverly Copland, who thought that I had the potential to complete this project and who eagerly gave me tons of strong support in the initial and ongoing book development phases.

Laurie Muench, who picked up the ball in the middle of manuscript preparation and persisted with me through the process to completion of book publication. The response "OK... when *can* I expect it?" provided silent encouragement and sometimes comic relief when my mental and physical energies ran quite low. Laurie's thoughtfulness and guidance to help me set priorities were invaluable! I am very grateful and fortunate to work with Laurie.

Suzi Epstein, who was full of enthusiasm and total support from the birth of the idea for a nursing review series to the final publication of the books. Suzi's creativity and suggestions provided essential building blocks in the overall development of the series.

My *coauthors,* for their enormous efforts to produce manuscript content in a short period of time. Their nursing expertise was helpful for the development of the unique aspects of each book.

My wonderful husband, *Dan,* for his patience, humor, support, and love. His faith in my abilities has sustained my energies and maintained my sense of self.

My parents, *Joseph and Mildred Demaske,* for their love, encouragement, and prayers.

Paulette D. Rollant

ACKNOWLEDGMENTS

There are many people I wish to thank for helping to make this a comprehensive, concise, and contemporary nursing review book.

First, I would like to extend a sincere thank you to a friend and colleague, *Denise McCann,* who offered me the support and encouragement needed to initiate the process of writing this book.

Members of the Department of Nursing and the division of Clinical Resource and Development at St. Joseph's Hospital Health Network in Syracuse, New York, were a daily inspiration to continue the process.

Mary Sue Stever and my sister, *Wendy Gratien,* spent many hours typing and retyping the manuscript as well as offering helpful editorial comments.

I would like to lovingly thank my mother, *Bernice Bramley,* and my sons, *Bruce* and *Brian,* for their love and patience over the last year.

Finally, I would like to acknowledge my deceased father, *Amos Bramley,* for encouraging me to always strive for excellence.

Denise Deppoliti

CONTENTS

HOW CAN I USE THIS BOOK?

This book is designed to work for you—at your convenience. Read the following guidelines first to help save you time and energy during test preparation. The chapters are designed for short, quick intervals of review. Carry this book with you to catch the times when you are stuck and have nothing to do.

The directions will help you to:
  ▼ **Maximize your individual performance in review and testing situations.**
  ▼ **Identify your personal priorities in preparation for testing.**
  ▼ **Sharpen your thinking and discrimination skills for testing.**

DIRECTIONS ON HOW TO REVIEW

  I. Identify your routine for reviewing: the best days, the best time of day
      A. Write the days and times on the inside front cover of this book and on your personal calendar and the calendar at home. This communicates to your family or support systems that you will be unavailable to them at these times. It is also a nice reminder every week to yourself that this is important to you.
      B. Refer to section V for specific directions on how to develop your routine
  II. Scan the table of contents
      A. Put a check mark in front of the content with which you are comfortable
      B. Circle the content in which you think you are weak
      C. Prioritize the weak content with #1 being the weakest content area. Put these numbers in front of your circles.
      D. Prioritize the strongest content areas in the same manner
  III. When you are feeling a high-energy day
      A. Go to the #1 chapter of the weakest content area for review
  IV. When you are having a low-energy day
      A. Go to the #1 chapter of the strongest content area for review

V. General guidelines for the development of a routine for reviewing
  A. Develop a system of review that meets your needs
  B. Set aside time when you are least tired or stressed both mentally and physically
  C. Limit your review time to a maximum of 90 minutes for the most effective, efficient retention of reviewed content
  D. If possible, relax and take a nap after reviewing to further place the information into long term memory. Some research reveals that sleeping for 2 to 3 hours after studying results in a 70 to 80% retention rate of content into long term memory in contrast to 30 to 40% retention when you are active after studying.
  E. Use at least one relaxation technique *at the onset* and *at the end* of your review time. Deep breathing that is slow with a concentration on the air movement going in and out is one of the best ways to relax physically and mentally.
  F. Use at least one relaxation technique *during* the time you review.
  G. If your time is limited, use 10 to 15 minute intervals to review small portions of the content. For example, you may want to review the different aspects of hypertension in one study session.
  H. Use a theme per week or per day approach. For example, if there is enough time between your test and when you begin to study, every Monday review something on sodium from the book. Then at work find clients with sodium imbalances, review their charts, and discuss their situations with colleagues or with the clients' physicians. Continue with themes for the day such as:
     1. Tuesdays are potassium
     2. Wednesdays are calcium
     3. Thursdays are magnesium
     4. Fridays are acidosis situations
     5. Saturdays are alkalosis days
     6. Sundays are fun days. Don't forget to keep one day to relax and have fun. This allows your mind to work for retention and reorganization of the content that you reviewed during the week.
     7. Weekly themes also might be of help. Do one system per week such as pulmonary, endocrine and so forth.

DIRECTIONS ON HOW TO USE THIS BOOK FOR SUCCESS

I. Suggested study sequence #1 for each chapter
  A. Read the objectives
  B. Complete the key terms

    C. Complete the content review
    D. Complete the review questions
    E. Review the answers, rationales, test-taking tips

II. Suggested study sequence #2 for each chapter
    A. Complete the review questions
    B. Review the answers, rationales, test-taking tips
    C. Review the missed content areas
    D. Review the unfamiliar and the familiar content areas
    E. Complete the key terms
    F. Complete the objectives to evaluate your level of understanding

III. Suggested study sequence #3 *after* doing #1 or #2 suggested sequence
    A. Complete the comprehensive exam in the book
    B. Correct comprehensive exam answers with review of the rationales and test-taking tips
    C. List content areas missed, then cluster them in terms of similar content
    D. Prioritize these clusters with #1 being the least familiar content
    E. Review additional content as directed by the questions you missed

IV. Suggested study sequence #4 *before* doing #1 or #2 suggested sequence
    A. Complete the comprehensive exam in the book
    B. Correct comprehensive exam answers with review of the rationales and test-taking tips
    C. List content areas missed, then cluster them in terms of similar content
    D. Prioritize these clusters with #1 being the least familiar content
    E. Implement either sequence #1 or #2
    F. Complete the computer comprehensive exam. Note that even though the questions are the same as in the book, you should evaluate how your reading of the questions and options differed as related to perception and consistent ability to identify key words, terms, age, and developmental needs.
    G. Review content as needed and directed from your missed questions on your exam

V. Suggested techniques for use of the objectives during your review
    A. Read the objectives to have them guide you where to start
    B. Put a check next to the ones in which you feel the weakest
    C. Prioritize them with #1 being the weakest
    D. Review the weakest content first or on high-energy days
    E. Review the most familiar content last or on low-energy days

VI. Suggested techniques for the use of the key terms, the content review section, and the exams
    A. Key terms—suggested study techniques
        1. Use a 3 x 5 index card to cover the definitions of the key terms
        2. State your definition out loud

3. Uncover the definition and read the given definition out loud (speaking the content as well as seeing the content will enhance your retention)

4. Write key notes in terms of a few words on a 3 x 5 card for the information you have difficulty recalling

5. Carry the card with you for a few days to review this content again. Suggestion: put the card on your sunvisor in the car and review it at the stoplight or if stopped in traffic.

B. Content review—suggested study techniques
1. Use a 3 x 5 card to cover the content under a major heading
2. State out loud what 3 or 4 important aspects of the content under the major heading might be or ask yourself a few questions about that content heading. Try to state the items in order of priority.
3. Uncover the content under the major heading. Check your information against that given in the book. See what you forgot or added that may or may not be important.
4. Write key notes in terms of a few words on a 3 x 5 card for the information you have difficulty recalling
5. Carry the card with you for a few days to review this content again. Suggestion: carry the card with you to review whenever you get 5 to 10 minutes free.
6. When you practice prioritizing the content you will enhance your critical thinking skills

C. Exam review—suggested study techniques
1. For all tests read all the rationales and test-taking tips for missed and correct questions. These often contain pearls of wisdom on how to remember or get a better understanding of the content.
2. Remember to do a relaxation exercise before you begin your questions and repeat the exercise about every 25 questions
3. When you miss a question ask yourself
   a. Did I not know the content?
   b. Did I misread the question or option(s)?
4. If you miss questions because of a knowledge deficit
   a. Make a list on a 3 x 5 card for 3 to 4 days
   b. Group or cluster the content according to the steps in the nursing process, the content area, or a system
   c. Look up that content
   d. Do not look up content after every practice test. A better approach is to cluster the content and look it all up every

3 to 4 days. With this approach you will have better retention into long term memory and the best recall at a later time.

    e. Try to identify new ways to approach reading questions and their options

5. If you misread the question or the option(s)

    a. Try to identify what key words, timeframes, ages, and developmental stages that you may have overlooked

    b. Try to identify new ways to approach reading the questions and their options

    c. Practice, practice, and practice doing questions

    d. Practice, practice, and practice doing relaxation before you begin the practice exam, after every 10 to 20 questions, and then at the end of the exam to refresh your thinking and diminish your tenseness or tiredness.

6. Be sure to do a practice exam with the exact number of questions as your real exam. Note after this exam when you were the most tired, anxious, or nervous. Plan to do a relaxation exercise at these times during the real exam.

7. Your success is directly correlated to your degree of effort to review content as well as relax during the review and exam processes.

SUMMARY

It is hoped that after you have completed your review with the use of this book as your major tool that you have:

▼ Maximized your individual performance in review and testing situations.

▼ Identified your personal priorities in preparation for testing.

▼ Sharpened your thinking and discrimination skills for testing.

Let this book work for you to make it easy, enjoyable, and effective to review at times that are convenient for you. The short, condensed, and prioritized chapter content may spark new ways to develop your skills in critical thinking and content recall.

It is feedback from students, graduates, and practitioners in nursing that prompted the development and publication of this book. We welcome your comments. We wish you a successful career in the nursing profession and hope that *Mosby's Nursing Review Series* has made that success a little easier to obtain!

▼ ▼ ▼ ▼ ▼ ▼ ▼ ▼ ▼   ▼ ▼ ▼

Essential Elements for Nursing

STUDY OUTCOMES

After completing this chapter, the reader will be able to do the following:

▼ Identify essential elements common to all nursing specialties.
▼ Discuss the priority content for each essential element.
▼ Incorporate the essential elements into nursing practice.

KEY TERMS

Client education	Process of meeting the client's needs for the acquisition of skills, knowledge, or attitudes to deal with a pathological condition in the arenas of primary, secondary, or tertiary health promotion as based on the prior skills, knowledge, and attitudes of the client.
Nursing process	Process used as the basis of nursing practice. It includes five steps: (1) assess, (2) select nursing diagnosis, (3) plan, (4) intervene, and (5) evaluate.

CONTENT REVIEW

ESSENTIAL ELEMENTS IN NURSING

I. The essential elements
   A. Nursing process
   B. Client education

II. Nursing incorporates these common essential elements irrespective of the level, environment, or client population

III. The nursing process is the priority common thread throughout nursing practice

IV. Client education facilitates clients' behavior changes in areas of primary (preventive), secondary (early diagnosis), and tertiary (restorative, rehabilitative) health promotion

NURSING PROCESS

I. The nursing process has five steps
   A. Assess
   B. Select nursing diagnosis
   C. Plan
   D. Intervene
   E. Evaluate

1. Nurses follow the nursing process sequence in any initial client contact
2. Evaluation of the interventions occurs to determine effectiveness or ineffectiveness
3. If effective results, the client-nurse relationship either terminates or new priorities are set for new client problems
4. If ineffective results, nurses select the appropriate step(s); at this point in the evaluation process, the sequence of steps is a creative process by nurses as dictated by client need
5. If a client has unexpected changes during care, nurses typically do further assessment of the situation before implementing actions
6. Use of these steps is a dynamic, client-centered process
7. Communication is essential in all phases of the nursing process

II. The initial assessment process

A. Includes subjective and objective information
B. Subjective information: elicited by questions such as
   1. What is the one item that made you decide to seek help?
   2. What is your major problem today?
   3. When did this start? How long did it last? What relieved it?
   4. Do I need to know any other information that can help me better care for you?
C. Objective information: elicited through the senses
   1. Inspection: done initially for the client's respiratory rate, breathing effort, color, and position
   2. Inspection and touch: a handshake of the client elicits
      a. Demonstration of respect for the client; reduction of client's anxiety
      b. Level of consciousness and the motor ability/strength of client to initiate an appropriate response
      c. Pulse assessment for rate and regularity if two-handed technique is used
      d. Skin assessment for temperature, color, texture, and moisture
   3. Smell for odors: done simultaneously with inspection
   4. Hearing: asking the initial questions, then auscultating elicits
      a. Specific information about the client's perception of the problem
      b. Information about the client's emotional reaction to the situation by noting the tone and inflection of the speech
      c. Degree of influence from others based on whether they answer or clarify client's answers to questions

        d. Auscultation typically includes the lungs, heart sounds, bowel sounds, and then any vascular sounds such as the carotid arteries or arterio-venous (A-V) fistulas

     5. Touch: commonly the approaches to other touch techniques such as percussion or palpation are completed by starting with the problem system then moving to the respiratory, cardiac, and neurological systems followed by the other systems

D. In emergency situations, objective information may take precedent over subjective information

     1. Airway, breathing, and circulation, the ABCs, may dictate assessment priorities

     2. Deferment of the history and physical assessment of all body systems may take a secondary focus, with priority actions aiming to support the cardiac and respiratory systems

E. Subjective information is best obtained from the client, the primary source, or from secondary sources such as the caretaker, family, or friends

F. History can be obtained from prior documentation to expedite the initial contact and conserve client energy

G. Results of the client's assessment, act as the foundation for selecting priority nursing diagnoses and the development of an appropriate plan of care

H. In acute- and home-care settings, nurses may limit priorities to two nursing diagnoses for a more realistic, attainable, efficient, and effective approach to client care

III. The selection of nursing diagnoses

A. Nursing diagnoses

     1. Are clinical judgments about responses of an individual or family to actual or potential threats to health or life situations

     2. Provide the basis for the selection of nursing interventions or referrals to achieve positive outcomes for evaluation

     3. Are designed with a three-part statement; however, in clinical practice the first part is consistently used, but the other parts may not be required as part of the documentation

        a. The three parts, also referred to as the PES format, are

           (1) P = health problem, stated as a nursing problem

           (2) E = etiological or related factors

           (3) S = the defining characteristics or cluster of signs/symptoms as identified from the assessment data

        b. The words *related to* connect the health problem and the etiological factors

      c. The words *as manifested by* connect the etiological factors and the signs/symptoms

      d. Example: urinary elimination—altered *related to* loss of muscle tone *as manifested by* incontinence, nocturia, dribbling.

      e. A health problem may be an actual or risk for (formerly potential or high-risk) problem

  B. **Process to the selection of nursing diagnoses**

    1. Assessment data are analyzed and interpreted for priorities in relation to time, for an actual or risk for problem with respect to what interventions are accountable by nursing

      a. In acute care: what needs to be accomplished

        (1) In the next 30 to 60 minutes?

        (2) In the next 8 hours?

        (3) In the next 24 hours?

        (4) By discharge from the facility?

      b. In other settings such as clinic, home, and outpatient care

        (1) What was the priority in the last few visits?

        (2) What necessitated this visit?

        (3) What has changed to require a reorganization of the priorities?

    2. A diagnostic label is selected with or without the phrases *related to* and *as manifested by;* institutional documentation policies guide the specific format for each agency

    3. In most situations, one or two priority nursing diagnoses are appropriate

    4. The ABCs are appropriate to use as a guide for setting priorities

IV. The planning process

  A. **Blueprint for nursing actions, also called nursing orders or planned nursing interventions, which are**

    1. Based on the priorities collected or clustered from the assessment data

    2. Selected in reference to time and resources available

    3. Safe for the client and the nurse

    4. Commonly a combination of independent, interdependent, and dependent actions

  B. **Involves goal setting for achievement of client outcomes**

  C. **May be done cooperatively if client is able to participate**

  D. **Commonly involves some component of education for a client knowledge deficit**

  E. Commonly dictates client outcomes, which need to be
      1. Achieved in a set amount of time
      2. Objective
      3. Realistic
      4. Observable or measurable for changes in client's activity,
          behavior, or physical state
      5. Used as a standard of measure in the evaluation process
      6. Examples
          a. Client outcome: within 48 hours the client will sleep
              through the night without the need to void
          b. Planned interventions
              (1) Provide use of the bedside commode before bedtime
              (2) Give no liquids after 8:00 P.M.

V. The intervention process
  A. Actual execution of the planned nursing actions
  B. Incorporates supervision, coordination, or evaluation of the
      delivery of care
  C. Includes the recording and exchange of information among
      different disciplines

VI. The evaluation process
  A. Based on client outcomes as identified from the planning
      process
  B. Determination of the degree of effectiveness or
      ineffectiveness of the interventions taken to achieve the
      stated outcomes
  C. Ongoing throughout the client-nurse relationship
  D. Often performed concurrently with other phases of the
      nursing process rather than as a distinctly individual step
  E. May result in the client's reassessment to reorder priorities
      and set new outcomes, especially if the stated time frame
      has been exceeded
  F. Requires documentation of the date when revisement or
      resolution of the health problem occurred; may be
      documented as ongoing
  G. Requires timely, accurate, and objective documentation and
      communication
  H. Includes identification of the client's level of knowledge and
      degree of willingness to change behaviors, skills, knowledge,
      or attitudes in any of these areas
      1. Diet
      2. Activity

3. Environment
4. Equipment
5. Medications: knowledge of
   a. Expected side effects
   b. Side effects that are treatable
   c. Side effects to report to the physician and within what time frame
   d. Length for the course of treatment

CLIENT EDUCATION

I. Client education: the process
A. Integral part of nursing care on either a formal or informal basis
B. Incorporates the use of the nursing process
C. Requires the use of teaching and learning principles
D. Varies with clients according to their life experiences, present situation, and age
E. Includes six main steps
   1. Assessment of client education needs or wants
   2. Identification of priorities
   3. Identification of client goals or outcomes: what is needed
      a. Behavior changes
      b. Skill acquisition
      c. Cognitive or attitude changes
   4. Development of a teaching plan
      a. Development of learner objectives
      b. Determination of the content required for the given situation
      c. Determination of the resources and how to use them
         (1) Identify the available referral support agencies
         (2) Identify the materials available for teaching/learning activities
         (3) Investigate whether there is money available for materials, courses, transportation to and from education classes
         (4) Estimate the amount of time available versus the amount of time needed to implement the teaching plan
         (5) Decide whether the nurse will initiate and complete the education or refer to another support service for the education
      d. Determination of sequence and presentation approach of the content

5. Implementation of the teaching plan over a stated time frame
6. Evaluation of outcomes with revisions or reteaching as needed

II. Client assessments for education

A. Client's knowledge base. What does the client know? What does he or she want to know? Respect that some clients desire no information and document that response.
B. Readiness
  1. Emotional
     a. Which stage of loss does client exhibit?
        (1) Denial
        (2) Anger
        (3) Bargaining
        (4) Depression
        (5) Acceptance
     b. If clients are in denial or anger, education will probably be ineffective; document stage of loss
  2. Motivational: intrinsic motivation, stimulated from within the learner, is preferred to extrinsic motivation, stimulated from outside the learner
  3. Experiential climate
     a. Values associated with social roles
     b. Personal resources and support systems
        (1) Family, friends
        (2) Finances for medications, equipment
        (3) Environmental factors: indoor plumbing, electricity
        (4) Prior and current exposure to interactions with the healthcare system and providers
        (5) Availability of healthcare services, time versus distance with available transportation
     c. Developmental stage
  4. Physical
     a. Clinical status is stable or improved
     b. Functional abilities
        (1) Hearing, attention span, listening
        (2) Vision
        (3) Touch and manual dexterity
        (4) Reading, level of highest education
        (5) Endurance
        (6) Short-term memory
           (a) Limited in its capacity
           (b) Enhanced if distractions are avoided

(c) Enhanced if opportunities are given for repeating or rehearsing the information

(7) Long-term memory

    (a) Unlimited in its capacity and duration

    (b) Influenced by the rate at which new information is introduced: the best approach is to introduce one new item every 4 to 5 seconds

    (c) Enhanced by 20 to 90% if material is incorporated into a story or real-life situation

5. Signs of client's readiness

    a. Beginning behaviors of adaption to the original problem

    b. Exhibits awareness of the health problem and its implications

    c. Asks direct questions

    d. Presents clues that suggest client is seeking information

    e. Begins to ask questions about how to handle situations at home

    f. Indicators during a teaching session

        (1) Client is physically comfortable; basic needs are met

        (2) Client readily gives attention; eye contact is made

        (3) Client turns off television or asks visitors to leave

III. Special needs of clients for their education

A. Interventions for low-literacy clients

1. Give only simple (basic) information
2. Present no more than three new points at a given time
3. Give the most important information first and last
4. Sequence information in the way the client will use it
5. Give information the client can use immediately
6. Use the same words when meanings are the same (e.g., medicine or drug, not both words)
7. Use small, simple words and short sentences; introduce no more than five new words in one session
8. Present information at the fifth-grade level or lower
9. Be concrete and time specific. Example: take two pills at 4:00 P.M.
10. Ask the client to repeat the information or the skill
11. Use humor appropriately; be creative
12. Avoid long explanations
13. Reward frequently—even for small accomplishments

B. Interventions for older clients

1. Priority evaluations

    a. Establish the degree of functional losses

      b. Identify the degree of social support; lack of social support may be an important determinant in the decreased compliance of older adults

      c. Identify their habit structures

      d. Have an evaluation completed by social services or the business office for the availability of monies

2. Clients with impaired hearing
    a. Use low-pitched voice
    b. Face client when speaking
    c. Use clear, concise terms

3. Clients with impaired vision
    a. Use large print and a magnifying glass
    b. Black on white or black on yellow paper may be easier for the older clients to read
    c. Provide adequate lighting
    d. Have client use prescription glasses

4. Clients with limited endurance
    a. Keep sessions short (10 to 15 minutes)
    b. Schedule the teaching session at a time of day when clients are comfortable and their energy levels are higher
    c. Break down the information into small steps
    d. The initial session should have only survival-level information

5. Clients with memory loss
    a. Provide repeated exposure to same message
    b. Provide cues: visual, verbal, written
    c. Question frequently
    d. Use advanced organizers: "I'm going to tell you 2 ways to give your insulin," "I've told you how to give your insulin by using two methods."

IV. Learning theory

A. Learning theory for adults

1. Adult learner is defined as a self-directed, independent person who becomes ready to learn when the need to know or perform is experienced
2. Adult education is learner centered
3. Adult education is dynamic, interactive, and cooperative
4. The responsibility for success of adult learners is shared by all participants
5. Adult learners
    a. Like to participate in identification of their learning needs, formulation of learning objectives, and evaluation of learning

        b.   Expect a climate of mutual respect
        c.   Enter the learning situation with a life-centered, task-centered, or problem-centered approach
        d.   Are motivated internally to learn in order to increase self-esteem, self-confidence, or seek a better quality of life
        e.   See the educator as a facilitator rather than a director of the activity

B. Learning theory for children
1. Learning programs for children are more subject centered
2. Design of learning experiences is topic centered
3. Learning may be more of an external process with emphasis on externally sanctioned approvals for learning such as stars, happy-face stickers
4. Objective, content development, and evaluation process are teacher controlled

C. Factors that interfere with learning
1. Nervousness, anxiety, fear
2. Too much content at one session
3. Unfamiliar terms
4. Complexity of the task
5. Limited time with too much content, results in rushing
6. Background noise or other distractions
7. Fear of the task or information
8. Frequent interruptions
9. Inability of an educator to listen to the client
10. Absence of silence
11. Left-handed student's learning skills with right-handed educator
12. Client is not healthcare oriented; healthcare educator is
13. Stage of development; older adults may have the attitude that they have lived more or less successfully with their present habits and there is no reason to change now

V. Tools for teaching

A. Types of teaching
1. One to one
2. Group
    a.   Homogeneous clients for a topic
    b.   Heterogeneous clients for a topic
3. Programmed instruction
4. Guided independent study
5. Lecture
6. Role playing

      7. Simulation
      8. Case method
      9. Demonstration/return demonstration
     10. Computerized instruction

B. Media for teaching
    1. Printed materials: pamphlets, books, crossword puzzles, study guides
    2. Pictorial materials: coloring books, videotapes, cartoons, flowcharts, slides, posters, overhead transparencies, computer simulations
    3. Visual representations: models, actual equipment
    4. Auditory: lectures, paired and small-group discussion, one-to-one interaction, role playing, cassette tapes, simulations
    5. Tactile, kinesthetic: practice with real or simulated items, manipulating or constructing models, playing games, completing worksheets, drawing, preparing charts, bulletin boards, developing a calendar of activities

C. Factors to consider in the selection of media/support materials
    1. Items readily available within acceptable costs
    2. Suitability: for the purpose of the teaching, to the environment in which the teaching will take place, for the availability of ancillary equipment
    3. Language: appropriate, understandable, and useful to the audience
    4. Materials: accurate and relevant to the intended age group and culture
    5. Print size: readable for the intended age group
    6. Illustrations: accurate and related to the intended audience

D. Nurse as a tool of teaching: the nursing professional should
    1. Show interest, empathy, and enthusiasm
    2. Practice expert listening skills; listen between the lines not only to what clients say, but how they say it
    3. Note clients' verbal and nonverbal communication that occurs; be aware of your own communication style
    4. Take a break when the client indicates a need; vary the schedule
    5. Be creative
    6. Keep language simple
    7. Allow enough time for demonstrations and return demonstrations
    8. Summarize at the end with encouragement for any progress, no matter how small

E. Evaluation tips for achievement of education outcomes
    1. Evaluation is an ongoing process throughout the entire teaching session

2. If periodic reassessment of learning indicates no progress, try a different approach
3. Ask open-ended questions along with specific questions
4. Ask clients to evaluate themselves

F. **Intervention tips for different age groups**
1. Pediatrics: the play approach works best with dolls or models; coloring, comic, or storybooks
2. Teenagers and persons in their 20s: use peer speakers, entertainment, and peer groups and keep in mind that body image and independence are a priority for these age groups
3. Persons in their 30s to mid-40s: written materials work well with follow-up time to answer questions or clarify information
4. Persons from mid-40s to early 60s: a few long, single sessions to discuss how the effects of the health problem will interfere with attainment of or plans for lifelong goals
5. Persons over mid-60s: use short, frequent, one-to-one meetings with material in larger print and keep in mind that maintaining functional abilities is a priority

SUMMARY

A working knowledge of the content in Chapter 1, the essential elements for nursing, will enhance the application of the remainder of the content in the review series. Most nursing professionals incorporate the two elements into their practice, which is based on the changing needs of clients who pursue the acquisition of healthcare services and actions to prevent pathological deterioration of the body. The nursing process and client education are intertwined in the areas of primary (preventive), secondary (early diagnosis), and tertiary (restorative, rehabilitative) health promotion.

NANDA-APPROVED NURSING DIAGNOSES

Activity intolerance
Activity intolerance, risk for
Adaptive capacity, decreased: intracranial
Adjustment, impaired
Airway clearance, ineffective
Anxiety
Aspiration, risk for
Body-image disturbance
Body temperature, altered, risk for
Bowel incontinence

Breastfeeding, effective
Breastfeeding, ineffective
Breastfeeding, interrupted
Breathing pattern, ineffective
Cardiac output, decreased
Caregiver role strain
Caregiver role strain, risk for
Communication, impaired verbal
Community coping, ineffective
Community coping, potential for enhanced
Confusion, acute
Confusion, chronic
Constipation
Constipation, colonic
Constipation, perceived
Coping, defensive
Coping, family: potential for growth
Coping, ineffective family: compromised
Coping, ineffective family: disabling
Coping, ineffective individual
Decisional conflict (specify)
Denial, ineffective
Diarrhea
Disuse syndrome, risk for
Diversional activity deficit
Dysreflexia
Energy field disturbance
Environmental interpretation syndrome: impaired
Family processes, altered
Family processes, altered: alcoholism
Fatigue
Fear
Fluid volume deficit
Fluid volume deficit, risk for
Fluid volume excess
Gas exchange, impaired
Grieving, anticipatory
Grieving, dysfunctional
Growth and development, altered
Health maintenance, altered
Health-seeking behaviors (specify)
Home maintenance management, impaired

Hopelessness
Hyperthermia
Hypothermia
Incontinence, functional
Incontinence, reflex
Incontinence, stress
Incontinence, total
Incontinence, urge
Infant behavior, disorganized
Infant behavior, disorganized: risk for
Infant feeding pattern, ineffective
Infection, risk for
Injury, perioperative positioning: risk for
Injury, risk for
Knowledge deficit (specify)
Loneliness, risk for
Management of therapeutic regimen, community: ineffective
Management of therapeutic regimen, families: ineffective
Management of therapeutic regimen, individuals: effective
Management of therapeutic regimen, individuals: ineffective
Memory, impaired
Mobility, impaired physical
Noncompliance (specify)
Nutrition, altered: less than body requirements
Nutrition, altered: more than body requirements
Nutrition, altered: risk for more than body requirements
Oral mucous membrane, altered
Pain
Pain, chronic
Parent/infant/child attachment altered, risk for
Parental role conflict
Parenting, altered
Parenting, altered, risk for
Peripheral neurovascular dysfunction, risk for
Personal identity disturbance
Poisoning, risk for
Posttrauma response
Powerlessness
Protection, altered
Rape-trauma syndrome
Rape-trauma syndrome: compound reaction
Rape-trauma syndrome: silent reaction

Relocation stress syndrome
Role performance, altered
Self-care deficit, bathing/hygiene
Self-care deficit, dressing/grooming
Self-care deficit, feeding
Self-care deficit, toileting
Self-esteem disturbance
Self-esteem, chronic low
Self-esteem, situational low
Self-mutilation, risk for
Sensory/perceptual alterations (specify) (visual, auditory, kinesthetic,
    gustatory, tactile, olfactory)
Sexual dysfunction
Sexuality patterns, altered
Skin integrity, impaired
Skin integrity, impaired, risk for
Sleep pattern disturbance
Social interaction, impaired
Social isolation
Spiritual distress (distress of the human spirit)
Spiritual well-being, potential for enhanced
Suffocation, risk for
Swallowing, impaired
Thermoregulation, ineffective
Thought processes, altered
Tissue integrity, impaired
Tissue perfusion, altered (specify type) (renal, cerebral,
    cardiopulmonary, gastrointestinal, peripheral)
Trauma, risk for
Unilateral neglect
Urinary elimination, altered
Urinary retention
Ventilation, inability to sustain spontaneous
Ventilatory weaning process, dysfunctional
Violence, risk for: self-directed or directed at others

CHAPTER 2

Mental Health-Mental Disorder Continuum

STUDY OUTCOMES

After completing this chapter, the reader will be able to do the following:

- ▼ Define the concepts of mental health and mental disorder.
- ▼ Discuss personality characteristics of mentally healthy individuals.
- ▼ Discuss factors contributing to the development of a mental disorder.
- ▼ Describe tools used to categorize mental disorders.

KEY TERMS

Coping mechanisms	Strategies for dealing with stress in an effort to produce psychological equilibrium.
Defense mechanisms	Function of the ego. They are unconscious mechanisms that decrease anxiety caused by conflicts between the id and the superego. The use of defense mechanisms returns the individual to equilibrium. Defense mechanisms may be both healthy and pathological.
Mental disorder	Responses to stress that create problems in intrapersonal and interpersonal functioning in the here and now.
Mental health	Ability to effectively adapt to stress in the here and now.
Stress response	Body's physiological responses to a change or perceived threat.
Stressors	Perceived threats to psychological and physical well-being.
V-codes	Other conditions that may be a focus of clinical attention.

CONTENT REVIEW

I. Historical Development of Concepts

A. **Mental health versus a mental disorder**
1. Culturally determined
2. Relative to time and place
3. Diagnoses focus on defining mental disorder instead of mental health
4. Mental health defined in negative terms—absence of disorder
5. Vague and abstract concepts
6. Difficult to scientifically measure either
7. Clinical interpretations lead to judgments and values
8. Exist on a continuum and are constantly changing
9. Process of labeling or categorizing (diagnosis and symptom orientation)
10. Label of mental disorder often places person in dependent status and in sick role

B. **Factors influencing process**
1. Methods of data collection
2. Social class of interpreter
3. Ethnic background of interpreter

II. Characteristics of the mentally healthy individual (Table 2-1)

III. Characteristics of the individual with a mental disorder (Table 2-2)

IV. Predisposing factors to a mental disorder (Figure 2-1)
    A. Biological
        1. Genetic background
        2. Nutritional status
        3. General health status
        4. Exposure to environmental toxins
    B. Psychological
        1. Intelligence
        2. Verbal ability
        3. Personality type
        4. Self-concept
        5. Verbal skills
        6. Past experiences
    C. Sociocultural
        1. Age

Table 2-1. Mentally Healthy Individual

Factors	Characteristics
Personality characteristics	Accepts self Loves self Goal oriented Thinks and acts independently Aware of own strengths and weaknesses Able to work productively
Adaptations to stress	In control of self and environment a majority of the time Effective coping mechanisms
Interpersonal relationships	Able to accept others Able to love others Able to care for others Able to be loved
Perception of environment and reality	Positive perception Reality oriented Able to find meaning in life

Table 2-2. Individual with a Mental Disorder

Factors	Characteristics
Personality characteristics	Unaccepting of self Dislikes self Dependent on others for thoughts and actions Lacks direction in life Unrealistic perception of strengths and weaknesses Lacks productivity in lifestyle Difficulty in meeting needs
Adaptations to stress	Often feels out of control of self; related to feelings and actions Often feels lack of control over environmental factors Ineffective coping mechanisms
Interpersonal relationships	Unable to accept thoughts and feelings of others Unable to love others Unable to care for others Unable to feel loved by others
Perception of environment and reality	Negative perception of environment Thoughts and perceptions may not be reality based Unable to find meaning or purpose in life

2. Education
3. Income
4. Occupation
5. Culture
6. Religious beliefs
7. Social relationships
8. Gender

V. Evaluation of precipitating stressors

A. Describe nature of the stressors (may be perceived as positive or negative events)
   1. Biological
   2. Psychological
   3. Sociocultural

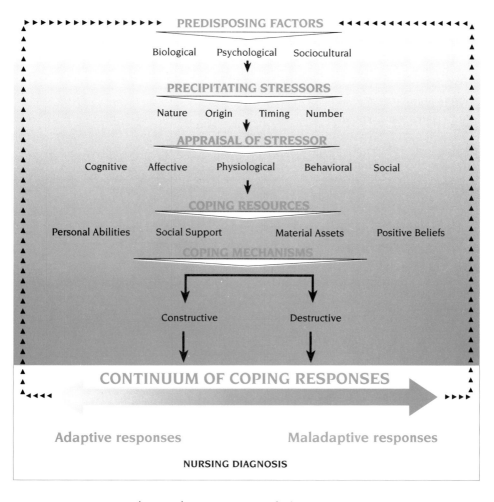

Figure 2-1. Biopsychosocial components of the stress adaptation model of psychiatric nursing care. (From Stuart G and Sundeen S: *Principles and practice of psychiatric nursing*, ed 5, St Louis, 1995, Mosby.)

B. Describe origin of the stressors
C. Timing
   1. When
   2. Duration
   3. Frequency
D. Number of stressors
   1. How many in period of time
   2. Dealing with more than one stressor at once may be overwhelming
   3. Types of stressors (Table 2-3 and Table 2-4)

Table 2-3. **Stressful Life Events**

Categories	Examples
Family	Child's going to college or moving back home after college
Work	Promotion
Education	Going back to school
Interpersonal	Divorce
Health	Being told one has a heart murmur
Financial	No cost-of-living increment
Legal	Being sued

VI. Primary appraisal: appraisal of the stressor (processing of the stressful situation)

A. Cognitive
   1. Evaluates potential damage according to situation's power to produce harm
   2. Threat of future harm
   3. Potential growth from the situation
B. Affective
   1. A "feeling state" in response to the stressor
      a. Anger
      b. Anxiety
      c. Fear
C. Physiological
   1. Autonomic nervous system response
   2. "Fight or flight"
D. Behavioral
   1. Reactive (defend against or flee the problem)
   2. Goal directed (solve the problem)
E. Social
   1. Seeks information about problem
   2. Determines factors that contribute to problem
   3. Compares strength of self to handle problem with that of others around them ("Do I need support?")

VII. Secondary appraisal: appraisal of coping resources (person's evaluation of own coping ability)

A. Cognitive
   1. What coping options are available?
   2. Will a strategy help?
   3. Can I utilize this method?

Table 2-4. Psychosocial and Environmental Problems

Problems Axis IV	Examples
Problems with primary support group	Death of a family member Health problems in the family Separation of parents Divorce Remarriage of parent Sexual or physical abuse Child neglect Birth of a sibling
Problems related to social environment	Death or loss of a friend Inadequate social support Living alone Difficulty with aculturation Retirement
Educational problems	Illiteracy Academic problems Discord with teachers or classmates
Occupational problems	Unemployment Threat of a job loss Difficult work conditions Job dissatisfaction Job change
Housing problems	Homelessness Inadequate housing Unsafe neighborhood
Economic problems	Extreme poverty Inadequate finances
Problems with access to health care services	Inadequate health care services Inadequate transportation to health care facilities Inadequate health insurance
Problems related to interaction with the legal system/crime	Arrest Incarceration Victim of crime
Other psychosocial and environmental problems	Disasters War Discord with caregivers Unavailability of social service agencies

From American Psychiatric Association: *Diagnostic and statistical manual of mental disorders,* 4th ed, Washington: DC, American Psychiatric Association, 1994

    B. Affective—expression of emotion
       1. Sadness
       2. Joy
       3. Fear
       4. Anger
       5. Acceptance
       6. Surprise
       7. Distrust
    C. Physiological—release of neuroendocrine substances
       1. Thyroid-stimulating hormones, T_3 and T_4; increase metabolism
       2. Vasopressin—antidiuretic hormone, ADH; increases water retention
       3. Prolactin
       4. Oxytocin
       5. Epinephrine—further initiates the stress response; stimulates breakdown of glucose stores
       6. Norepinephrine—causes vasoconstriction
       7. Insulin—facilitates the use of more glucose
    D. Behavioral
       1. Change the stressor
       2. Escape the stressor
       3. Acquire new abilities to change the stressor or change the reaction to the stressor
       4. Defend against an emotional response
       5. Adjust to the stressor
    E. Social—evaluation of available support (adapted from Stuart and Sundeen, 1991)

VIII. Types of coping mechanisms

    A. Coping mechanism—any effort to decrease the stress response, such as jogging, listening to music, and walking
    B. Task-oriented—direct problem solving. Example: "I failed a test; I will study differently next time."
    C. Defense-oriented—regulating response to protect self. Example: "I wasn't late; you expected me to be early."
    D. Either constructive or destructive in nature. Example: jogging versus drinking alcoholic beverages.
    E. Destructive coping mechanisms often cause a mental disorder, since the problem is avoided. Neurotic or psychotic behaviors typically result.

IX. Levels of dysfunctional coping in the mental disorder continuum

A. Neurotic (types and examples)
   1. A symptom or group of symptoms that is distressing and is recognized as unacceptable or alien to the individual. Example: having to perform an action repeatedly.
   2. Reality testing is grossly intact: aware of time, place, person, unlike psychotic coping
   3. Behavior does not actively violate gross social norms; it is not harmful to other people. Example: stirring coffee 20 times before drinking.
   4. The neurotic disturbance is relatively enduring or recurrent without treatment, and it is not limited to a transitory reaction to stressors—symptoms last for months or even years
   5. There is no measurable organic cause or factor—no physical reason for the behavior

B. Psychotic (types and examples)
   1. A severe mood disorder—so depressed that a person is unable get out of bed
   2. Regressive behavior—lying in bed in a fetal position
   3. Personality disintegration—unaware of self, "who they are" or group identity
   4. A significant reduction in level of awareness—may be mute and immobile
   5. Great difficulty in functioning adequately—may not be able to go to school or work
   6. Gross impairment in reality testing—believe that they are Jesus Christ or the president of the United States (Stuart and Sundeen, 1991)

X. DSM IV—Diagnostic and statistical manual of mental disorders of the American Psychiatric Association

A. Medical diagnoses are stated and classified
B. Names of various disorders are listed
C. Description of diagnostic criteria is presented
D. Test for reliability is reported
E. Multiaxial system
   1. Axis I—clinical disorders and V-codes, other conditions that may be a focus of clinical attention
   2. Axis II—personality disorders and mental retardation
   3. Axis III—general medical conditions
   4. Axis IV—psychosocial and environmental problems (see Table 2-4)
   5. Axis V—global assessment of functioning (Table 2-5)

Table 2-5. Global Assessment of Functioning (GAF) Scale

Code (Note: Use intermediate codes when appropriate, e.g., 45, 68, 72.)

Consider psychological, social, and occupational functioning on a hypothetical continuum of mental health–illness. Do not include impairment in functioning due to physical (or environmental) limitations.

100-91	Superior functioning in a wide range of activities, life's problems never seem to get out of hand, is sought out by others because of his or her many positive qualities. No symptoms.
90-81	Absent or minimal symptoms (e.g., mild anxiety before an exam), good functioning in all areas, interested and involved in a wide range of activities, socially effective, generally satisfied with life, no more than everyday problems or concerns (e.g., an occasional argument with family members).
80-71	If symptoms are present, they are transient and expectable reactions to psychosocial stressors (e.g., difficulty concentrating after family argument); no more than slight impairment in social, occupational, or school functioning (e.g., temporarily falling behind in schoolwork).
70-61	Some mild symptoms (e.g., depressed mood and mild insomnia) OR some difficulty in social, occupational, or school functioning (e.g., occasional truancy, or theft within the household), but generally functioning pretty well, has some meaningful interpersonal relationships.
60-51	Moderate symptoms (e.g., flat affect and circumstantial speech, occasional panic attacks) OR moderate difficulty in social, occupational, or school functioning (e.g., few friends, conflicts with peers or co-workers).
50-41	Serious symptoms (e.g., suicidal ideation, severe obsessional rituals, frequent shoplifting) OR any serious impairment in social, occupational, or school functioning (e.g., no friends, unable to keep a job).
40-31	Some impairment in reality testing or communication (e.g., speech is at times illogical, obscure, or irrelevant) OR major impairment in several areas, such as work or school, family relations, judgment, thinking, or mood (e.g., depressed man avoids friends, neglects family, and is unable to work; child frequently beats up younger children, is defiant at home, and is failing at school).
30-21	Behavior is considerably influenced by delusions or hallucinations OR serious impairment in communication or judgment (e.g., sometimes incoherent, acts grossly inappropriately, suicidal preoccupation) OR inability to function in almost all areas (e.g., stays in bed all day; no job, home, or friends).

Table 2-5. Global Assessment of Functioning (GAF) Scale—cont'd

Code (Note: Use intermediate codes when appropriate, e.g., 45, 68, 72.)

20-11	Some danger of hurting self or others (e.g., suicide attempts without clear expectation of death; frequently violent; manic excitement) OR occasionally fails to maintain minimal personal hygiene (e.g., smears feces) OR gross impairment in communication (e.g., largely incoherent or mute).
10-1	Persistent danger of severely hurting self or others (e.g., recurrent violence) OR persistent inability to maintain minimal personal hygeine OR serious suicidal act with clear expectation of death.
0	Inadequate information.

The rating of overall psychological functioning on a scale of 0-100 was operationalized by Luborsky in the Health-Sickness Rating Scale (Luborsky L: "Clinicians' Judgements of Mental Health." *Archives of General Psychiatry* 7:407-417, 1962). Spitzer and colleagues developed a revision of the Health-Sickness Rating Scale called the Global Assessment Scale (GAS) (Endicott J, Spitzer RL, Fleiss JL, Cohen J: "The Global Assessment Scale: A Procedure for Measuring Overall Severity of Psychiatric Disturbance." *Archives of General Psychiatry* 33:776-771, 1976). A modified version of the GAS was included in DSM-III-R as the Global Assessment of Functioning (GAF) Scale.
(American Psychiatric Association: *Diagnostic and Statistical Manual of Mental Disorders,* 4th ed, Washington, DC, 1994, American Psychiatric Association)

    F. DSM IV is the major tool used professionally in the United States to categorize mental disorders

XI. Guideline for the selection of nursing diagnoses
    A. Actual or potential responses to stressors are the focuses
    B. Statement of client's problem with a related statement of findings for the structure
    C. The problem must be one for which nursing interventions are appropriate and legal
    D. Nurses most often utilize axes IV and V in identifying problem areas for nursing interventions

REVIEW QUESTIONS

1. The nurse is leading a group session with 10 clients. When observing behavior, the nurse should remember that behavioral symptoms of these clients
    a. Have meaning
    b. Are purposeful
    c. Are easily understood
    d. Are intentional

2. A client has been in the hospital for 7 days from complications of an acute myocardial infarction and left-sided heart failure. The client's history includes diabetes for the past 10 years and occasional periods of paranoia. As the nurse enters the room, the client shouts, "Get out! Don't touch me! You don't know what you are doing!" When dealing with this angry, agitated client, initially it is most important for the nurse to respond by
    a. Leaving the client alone
    b. Using statements of authority
    c. Seeking assistance immediately
    d. Avoiding internalization of the client's anger

3. The primary goal in the treatment of the psychiatric client is to
    a. Relieve psychiatric symptoms
    b. Discharge the client to home as soon as possible
    c. Prevent the client from becoming psychotic
    d. Assist the client to become a better-adjusted individual

4. The DSM IV is a tool utilized for diagnosis in mental health settings. This multiaxial system includes
    a. Nursing and medical diagnoses
    b. Frameworks of specific theories
    c. Assessments for several areas of functioning
    d. Specific critical pathways

5. Characteristics of a mentally healthy individual include
    a. A difficulty in meeting needs
    b. A negative perception of the environment
    c. A frequent feeling of lack of control over the environment
    d. An awareness of needs for improvement

ANSWERS, RATIONALES, AND TEST-TAKING TIPS

Rationales	Test-Taking Tips

1. **Correct answer: a**

   Behavior, normal or abnormal, is reflective and interpretive of any individual's thoughts and actions. Not all behavior is purposeful or intentional. Some behaviors are spontaneous, with the purpose or intention identified later. Some behaviors are easily understood, and others are more complex, with the understanding of them taking months or years.

   If you have no idea of the correct answer, cluster options *b* and *c* under the umbrella of behaviors that are thought of before being carried out. Eliminate these options, since some behavioral symptoms may be spontaneous. Delete option *c* with the use of common sense reasoning that behaviors are not always easily understood. Select option *a*.

2. **Correct answer: d**

   Often, with agitated clients, anger is misplaced and not directed toward any particular person. Nurses should be first aware of their own reactions to threatening situations or anger. Next they should be able to distance themselves from the clients' actions, words, and feelings and not be affected by them. Avoidance is a nontherapeutic response where nurses may refuse to recognize or deal with the anger; this leaves the clients feeling more frustrated and then resorting to withdrawal. Use of an authority statement, a nontherapeutic response, in an attempt to provide nursing care may deteriorate into a

   If you have no idea of the correct answer, cluster options *a, b* and *c* under "actions of the nurse." Option *d* is a nurse's mental activity, with an approach of the nurse to respond rather than to react to the client's behavior.

power struggle between the client and the nurse. No information is given to support the selection of seeking assistance.

3. Correct answer: d

The primary treatment goal is for the psychiatric client to be better adjusted to meet the demands of daily life. A psychiatric client may not be symptom free. A discharge to the client's home is dependent on the individual client's progress as based on a critical pathway. In option *c* note that not all psychiatric clients have the risk of becoming psychotic.

If you have no idea of the correct answer, note that the question is general, without any specific information. Therefore a more general option *d*, will be best. Options *a, b,* and *c* are more specific; they address specific focuses of symptoms, psychotic behavior, and discharge.

4. Correct answer: c

The multiaxial system assesses five areas: clinical syndromes, developmental/personality disorders, physical disorders/conditions, severity of psychosocial stressors, and global functional assessment. This system classifies mental illness, as well as presents guidelines and diagnostic criteria for various mental disorders. From these guidelines, healthcare practitioners state nursing or medical diagnoses or develop specific critical pathways. Frameworks of specific theories are best found in textbooks.

Use the following approach if you have no idea of the correct answer. Reread the question to note that it is asking about a tool used for "diagnosis." This is a clue to associate that, before making a diagnosis, one usually collects assessment information. Reread the options and select *c,* since it includes "assessments . . . of functioning."

5. **Correct answer: d**

Mentally healthy individuals are aware of their needs and realize that improvement of self is an ongoing process. The characteristics in options *a, b,* and *c* describe individuals with mental disorders.

If you have no idea of the correct answer, use the cluster approach for options *a, b,* and *c* which are negative statements.

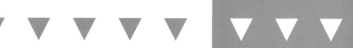

Defense
Mechanisms

STUDY OUTCOMES

After completing this chapter, the reader will be able to do
the following:

▼ Discuss the role of defense mechanisms in the reduction of anxiety.

▼ Define the most common defense mechanisms.

▼ Identify life examples of each defense mechanism.

KEY TERMS

Anxiety	A response to a stressor that cannot be directly observed. It is a vague sense of impending doom that seems to have no basis in reality. It is contagious. There are four levels of anxiety.
Coping mechanisms	Are based on a conscious acknowledgement that a problem exists. The individual engages in reality-oriented problem-solving activities designed to reduce tension (Taylor, 1993).
Ego defense mechanisms	A function of the ego. They are unconscious mechanisms that decrease anxiety caused by conflicts between the id and the superego. The use of defense mechanisms returns the individual to equilibrium and their use may be both healthy and pathological.
Fear	Response to a real external stressor that is threatening to self.
Pathological defense mechanisms	Avoidance of the problem. They interfere with reality and interpersonal relationships and distort basic personality.

CONTENT REVIEW

I. Defense mechanisms (Table 3-1)
   A. Are unconscious
   B. Decrease anxiety
   C. Are a protective response to conflict between id and superego
   D. Use psychic energy
   E. Eighteen types of ego defense mechanisms (Table 3-2)
      1. Compensation
         a. Perceived inadequacy or weakness
         b. Emphasizes personal attribute to make up for this perception
         c. Gains social approval
         d. Often a result of guilt or inferiority
      2. Conversion
         a. Expression of emotional conflicts through physical symptoms
         b. Repression is utilized first
         c. Person is unaware of connection between symptoms and conflict

Table 3-1. Comparison of Effective and Ineffective Coping Mechanisms; Nonpathological and Pathological Defense Mechanisms

Mechanisms	Purpose	Process	Outcome
Effective coping mechanisms	Reduce tension Solve problems	Conscious process Directly confront problem	Tension is reduced Problem is resolved
Ineffective coping mechanisms	Reduce tension	Conscious process Indirectly confront problem Avoid problem	Tension may be temporarily decreased but reappears later Problem is still present
Nonpathological defense mechanisms	Decrease anxiety Resolve conflict between the id and the superego	Unconscious process	Return individual to equilibrium
Pathological defense mechanisms	Decrease anxiety Resolve conflict between the id and the superego	Unconscious process Avoid problem	Individual does not return to equilibrium; has disruptions in interpersonal relationships and perception of reality, along with distortion of personality

Table 3-2. Ego Defense Mechanisms

Defense Mechanism	Example
Compensation	A physically small teenage male who does poorly in athletic competition is on the honor roll.
Conversion	A young woman ambivalent about her upcoming marriage wakes up paralyzed the morning of her wedding.
Denial	A diabetic does not take his insulin and goes out for a hot fudge sundae.
Displacement	A man who was fired from his job goes home and kicks his dog.
Dissociation	A young girl who was sexually abused by her father has no recollection of this until, as an adult, she is raped from the waist down.
Fixation	A young man smokes three packs of cigarettes a day and weighs 300 pounds.
Identification	A girl dresses like her favorite female teacher.
Intellectualization	A man who has recently been diagnosed with cancer discusses his various treatment options but is unable to connect with a feeling about his diagnosis.
Introjection	A woman with bipolar disorder stabs herself in the abdomen to kill her mother, who she believes to be in her stomach.
Isolation	A mother talks unemotionally about her child who was stillborn yesterday.
Projection	A young boy who unconsciously dislikes himself believes that it is his classmates who dislike him.
Rationalization	"I would have done better on the test if the teacher had stressed the right information."
Reaction formation	A man who is unaware or unconscious of the fact that he dislikes his mother-in-law is very nice to her and talks about how wonderful she is.
Regression	When 6-year-old Tommy's sister is born, he begins wetting his pants after 3 years of being out of diapers.
Repression	A man is unable to remember the car accident he was in last week in which his brother was killed.
Sublimation	An unmarried woman who desires to have children becomes a grammar school teacher.
Symbolization	A man who questions his masculinity buys guns and is constantly at target practice.
Undoing	A man who had a fight with his wife last week decides to send her a dozen roses to tell her how much he loves her.

    d. Symptom directly relates to the conflict

    e. Symptom distracts from the real problem

3. Denial

    a. Defends against onset of massive anxiety

    b. Person is not aware of an event or feeling in the here and now

    c. Person acts as if the event or feeling did not exist

4. Displacement

    a. Feelings toward one person are directed to another

    b. Substitute is a safer object

    c. Often the feeling is negative, such as anger

5. Dissociation

    a. Separation or splitting of effect from an idea, situation, or object

    b. Walling off of an anxiety-provoking event or period of time from the conscious mind

    c. The portion of personality associated with stress is kept out of awareness

6. Fixation

    a. Certain aspects of emotional development stop

    b. Further development is blocked

    c. Result of difficulty in a phase of development

7. Identification

    a. Normal process of development

    b. Take on admired attributes of others

    c. Integrate attributes into personality

    d. Defends against feelings of inadequacy by exhibiting attributes of admired person

8. Intellectualization

    a. Thinking is disconnected from feelings

    b. Situations are dealt with at a cognitive level

    c. Emotional aspect is avoided or ignored

9. Introjection

    a. Replacement of personality or parts of personality

    b. Symbolic swallowing of an aspect of another person

    c. Precipitated by a real or perceived loss of this person

    d. May lose own personality in the process

10. Isolation

    a. Feeling is disconnected from the experience

    b. Can recall or experience the event without the anxiety

11. Projection

    a. Transfer own unacceptable ideas, thoughts, and feelings onto another person

      b. Own thoughts are unacceptable or cause anxiety

      c. Often used by the mentally ill—own self-hate projected to others ("I don't hate myself; they hate me")

12. Rationalization

      a. Attempt to make one's behavior acceptable to self and others

      b. Sense of guilt about thoughts or behaviors

      c. Saving face

      d. Not intentionally being false

      e. Assists in avoiding reality

13. Reaction formation

      a. Unconscious feelings or wishes are unacceptable

      b. Act in a way that is opposite to the true feeling or wish

      c. Often very friendly or polite to compensate for anger

14. Regression

      a. Situation cannot get solved through usual behaviors

      b. Resort to behaviors from earlier stages

      c. Behaviors appropriate to earlier development stages

      d. Often dependent on others

15. Repression

      a. Painful experiences, thoughts, or impulses are forgotten

      b. Takes much psychic energy to keep unconscious

      c. May escape into physical symptoms or anxiety

      d. Primary defense—operates as a part of all other defenses

16. Sublimation

      a. Anxiety caused by primitive impulses is redirected into socially acceptable behaviors

      b. Often a positive response to anxiety

      c. Responsible for creative behavior

17. Symbolization

      a. Idea or object is substituted for one that is anxiety producing

      b. Often appear in dreams or fantasies

      c. Instinctual desires often appear through symbols

18. Undoing

      a. Engages in behavior to cancel out an unacceptable behavior, thought, or feeling

      b. Aware of behavior but not purpose

      c. May be basis for compulsive behavior

      d. Behavior is often repetitive

REVIEW QUESTIONS

1. A nursing student is reprimanded by the clinical instructor. The student comes homes and kicks the family dog. This illustrates
   a. Identification
   b. Projection
   c. Repression
   d. Displacement

2. A client has been admitted with an MI. The client talks about adjustments that must be made after discharge. The client states, "I will give up certain activities because they don't matter anyway." This is an example of
   a. Denial
   b. Displacement
   c. Regression
   d. Rationalization

3. A client experienced a right-sided CVA two weeks ago. During one of the client's home visits, a daughter comments that the client insists on feeding and dressing as if nothing had happened. This client is coping by
   a. Intellectualization
   b. Isolation
   c. Repression
   d. Denial

4. The wife of a fundamentalist minister occasionally daydreams of being a rock star. This is an example of
   a. Role reversal
   b. Fantasy
   c. Symbolization
   d. Compensation

5. Which situation best exemplifies undoing?
   a. A mother talks unemotionally about a stillborn child of yesterday
   b. A student says, "I would have a higher grade if the professor had stressed the essential information"
   c. A husband sends flowers to his wife a week after a fight to tell her how much he loves her
   d. A young girl who unconsciously dislikes herself believes that her classmates dislike her

ANSWERS, RATIONALES, AND TEST-TAKING TIPS

Rationales	Test-Taking Tips

1. Correct answer: d

Displacement is the discharging of pent-up emotions to a less threatening object or person. Identification, a normal process of development, is the taking on of admired attributes of others or attempting to pattern or resemble the personality of an admired, idealized person. Projection is the transfer of one's own unacceptable ideas, thoughts, or feelings onto another person. Repression is a primary defense that operates as a part of all other defenses; it is an unconscious process where painful experiences, thoughts, or impulses are forgotten.

Remember that displacement involves negative feeling toward a safer object or person.

2. Correct answer: d

Rationalization is an attempt to prove one's feelings are justifiable and acceptable to self and others. Denial defends against the onset of massive anxiety where the person acts as if the event or feeling did not exist. In regression the client resorts to behaviors of earlier developmental stages when a situation cannot get resolved through usual behaviors.

If you have no idea of the correct response, use common sense to eliminate options *a, b,* and *c,* since there is no information such as a change of the subject to indicate denial; nothing is stated to reflect displacement of feeling to a safer object; and nothing to indicate that the client has returned to behaviors of an earlier stage. Select option *d.*

3. **Correct answer: d**

   Denial is the unconscious refusal to admit to unacceptable behaviors or ideas. In intellectualization, thinking is disconnected from feelings; the emotional aspect is avoided or ignored. In isolation a client can recall or experience an event without the anxiety. Repression is the unconscious or involuntary forgetting of painful events and conflicts.

   The clue in the stem are the words "as if nothing happened." This is most indicative of denial. For your exam preparation, you may want to practice intellectualization (to ignore emotions tied to exams) and isolation (to experience the exam process without anxiety).

4. **Correct answer: b**

   Fantasy is the unconscious retreat into daydreams and imagination to escape realistic problems or to avoid conflict. Role reversal is the use of role playing to achieve an attitude change or self-awareness. Symbolization is substituting an idea or object for repressed thoughts, feelings, or impulses; often these appear in dreams or fantasies. Compensation emphasizes a personal attribute to make up for a perceived inadequacy.

   Use logic to associate "daydream" with "fantasy."

5. **Correct answer: c**

   Option *a* represents isolation. Option *b* describes rationalization. Option *d* illustrates projection.

   If you have no idea of the correct answer, the common sense approach is to identify which action is described to most likely "make up for a prior action."

Interdisciplinary Mental Health Treatment Team; Role of the Nurse

STUDY OUTCOMES

After completing this chapter, the reader will be able to do the following:

▼ Define psychiatric nursing.

▼ Distinguish between primary, secondary, and tertiary prevention.

▼ Identify the roles of various members of the interdisciplinary treatment team.

▼ Discuss the nature and the setting of psychiatric nursing practice.

▼ Discuss the application of the American Nurses' Association Standards of Psychiatric-Mental Health Nursing Practice.

▼ Apply the nursing process in caring for a psychiatric client.

KEY TERMS

Interdisciplinary	Members of different disciplines who treat the client interdependently, based on separate and distinct roles of each team member (Table 4-1).
Multidisciplinary	Members of different disciplines who each provide specific services to the client.
Unidisciplinary	All team members of the same discipline.

CONTENT REVIEW

I. Psychiatric nursing practice
A. Interpersonal approach
B. Client classifications
   1. Individual
   2. Family
   3. Group
   4. Community
C. Purposeful use of self to achieve outcomes
D. Concerned with promotion of mental health
E. Sources of knowledge
   1. Nursing science
   2. Psychosocial science
   3. Biophysical science
   4. Theories of personality
F. Individuals interact with the environment
G. Practice settings
   1. Psychiatric hospitals
   2. Community mental health centers
   3. General hospitals
   4. Community health agencies
   5. Outpatient clinics
   6. Homes
   7. Schools
   8. Prisons
   9. Health maintenance organizations
   10. Crisis care units
   11. Day care centers
   12. Night care centers
   13. Physician offices

Table 4-1. Members of the Mental Health Team

Team Member	Educational Preparation	Function on the Team
Psychiatric nurse	RN (diploma), AA, BS; advanced preparation at the master's level for independent practice	Provides environmental management and 24-hour care Carries out individual, family, and group psychotherapy and coordinates team activities Supervises technicians or psychiatric assistants Plays primary, secondary, and tertiary roles in the community
Clinical nurse specialist (CNS)	Master's degree in psychiatric mental health nursing	Advanced nurse practitioner who provides individual, group, and family psychotherapy Includes function of role model to other staff and clients, as well as staff educator, researcher, clinical expert, and consultant

Nurse practitioner (NP)	Certificate program post RN
	American Nurses Credentialing Center certification as NP—higher level of credentialing not presently required to be a NP
	Trend moving toward requirement of a master's degree. The requirements may vary from state to state.
		Work in conjunction with physicians/psychiatrists to
		▶ Treat common health problems
		▶ Diagnose common disease processes
		Provides
		  ▶ Health counseling
		  ▶ Health promotion
		  ▶ Individual and family therapy per state protocol
		Manages chronic medical problems
		Monitors effectiveness and side effects of psychotropic medications
		Prescriptive privileges if certified per state protocol
		May be elegible for third party reimbursement in some states

Continued.

Table 4-1. Members of the Mental Health Team—cont'd

Team Member	Educational Preparation	Function on the Team
Psychiatrist	MD/DO with residency in psychiatry	Physician who specializes in the treatment of mental disorders Has both administrative and care-planning responsibilities; diagnostic and medical functions are the psychiatrist's main tasks
Clinical psychologist	PhD in clinical psychology	Specializes in the study of mental processes and treatment of mental disorders Utilizes diagnostic testing to assist the team in differentiating the causative factors in client's behavior Treats clients, by use of both individual and group methods
Psychiatric social worker	Master's degree in social work (MSW)	Evaluates families; studies the environment and social causes of the client's illness Practices family therapy as a natural outcome of assessment
Psychiatric assistant or technician	High school education, special on-job training in setting of employment	Works under the direct supervision of a professional nurse Assists nurses in providing for the basic needs of clients Carries out nursing functions, including maintenance of a therapeutic environment Supervises leisure activities Assists with individual and group psychotherapy

Occupational therapist	Advanced degree in occupational therapy	Assesses client's skills for rehabilitative planning Encourage clients to perform useful tasks Provides socialization therapy and vocational retraining
Art therapist	Advanced degree and specialized training in art therapy	Utilizes procedures that make use of spontaneous creative works of the client Works with groups, encouraging members to make and analyze drawings, which are often expressions of their underlying problems Acts as adjunct to a mental health team in diagnosis and treatment of children
Recreational therapist	Advanced degree and specialized training in recreational therapy	Provides leisure activities for clients Teaches hospitalized clients useful pastimes, which can be utilized when they return to the community Participates in pet therapy, psychodrama, poetry, and music therapy
Dietitian	Advanced degree and specialized training in dietetics	Provides for the preparation of attractive, nourishing meals for clients Is involved in direct treatment of such food-related illnesses as anorexia nervosa, bulimia, and pica

H. **Roles of the psychiatric nurse**
1. Staff nurses
2. Administrators
3. Consultants
4. In-service educators
5. Clinical practitioners
6. Client educators

I. **Functions of the psychiatric nurse**
1. Primary prevention
   a. Stresses community's influence
   b. Changes causative factors before they can do harm
   c. Results of interventions precede a disease process
   d. Intervenes for health promotion
   e. Intervenes for illness prevention
   f. Provides health teaching
   g. Actions aimed at improving living conditions
   h. Completes assessments of potential stressors and life changes
   i. Coordinates/implements community education related to mental health
2. Secondary prevention
   a. Reduces mental illness by early detection and treatment
   b. Completes intake screening and evaluation
   c. Conducts home visits
   d. Provides emergency treatment
   e. Provides a therapeutic milieu
   f. Supervises clients receiving medication
   g. Participates in suicide prevention
   h. Participates in crisis intervention
   i. Conducts psychotherapy—individual, family, group
3. Tertiary prevention
   a. Reduces residual impairment or disability
   b. Makes referrals to the following:
      (1) Vocational training and rehabilitation
      (2) Aftercare programs and/or partial hospitalization options (Stuart G and Sundeen S, 1991)

Table 4-2. **Nursing Process Sample**

Assessment data

▼ Believes that all people in the environment are spies
▼ Believes he is in prison. Perceives others' comments as hostile or sexual overtures

Nursing diagnosis

▼ Altered thought process related to anxiety and decreased self-esteem

Outcome criteria

▼ Demonstrates reality based thinking in verbal and nonverbal behavior
▼ Verbally states he is in the hospital; no longer believes others to be spies

Nursing interventions in order of action

▼ Approach in slow, calm, matter-of-fact manner
▼ Assess client's ability to think logically
▼ Refrain from touching the client, particularly when client is out of contact with reality
▼ Use simple, concrete sentences
▼ Do not argue with the client about delusions
▼ Distract the client from delusions by engaging client in other activities
▼ Focus on feelings evoked by the delusions rather than on the delusion itself
▼ Encourage client to discuss experiences that occurred before the onset of the delusion
▼ Do not ask questions about the content of the delusions

Evaluation

▼ Communicates thoughts and feelings in a coherent way
▼ Displays understandable verbal communication
▼ Exhibits awareness that the setting is in the hospital
▼ States that people are not spying on him and exhibits awareness of the various roles of the hospital staff

REVIEW QUESTIONS

1. In which type of meeting are client behaviors discussed individually, with decisions made about treatments?
   a. Group meetings
   b. Community meetings
   c. Team meetings
   d. Supervision meetings

2. What professional group more commonly assumes the leadership responsibility for team meetings?
   a. Nurses
   b. Social workers
   c. Psychiatrists
   d. Psychologists

3. Which activity of the psychiatric nurse is least likely associated with secondary prevention?
   a. Provides emergency treatment
   b. Completes intake screening
   c. Conducts home visits
   d. Provides health teaching

4. The primary role of the nurse in care of the psychiatric client is to
   a. Collaborate with other disciplines
   b. Conduct intake evaluations
   c. Coordinate client care
   d. Participate in the decision making

5. A newly admitted client to the psychiatric unit requires physical restraint for protection to self and the staff. The available staff consists of two licensed persons, a psychiatric technician, and a security staff member. Under the direct supervision of the registered nurse, what is the most appropriate use of the staff?
   a. Have the licensed staff restrain the client
   b. Have all staff restrain the client
   c. Direct the licensed staff and security to restrain the client
   d. Direct the technician and security to restrain the client

ANSWERS, RATIONALES, AND TEST-TAKING TIPS

Rationales	Test-Taking Tips

1. Correct answer: c

Team meetings include all disciplines: medicine, nursing, social work, and occupational/recreational therapy. The client's case is reviewed, and treatment goals are revised.

If you have no idea of the correct answer, first note that the question is specific about a client's behaviors. Then cluster options *a, b,* and *d* under the category of meetings with a general or global focus. Select option *c,* which may more likely reflect a meeting to focus on an individual.

2. Correct answer: a

Nursing more commonly assumes leadership for team meetings. When clients are admitted, nurses assume the therapist and client advocate roles, which allows for better representation of the client during team meetings.

Cluster options *b, c,* and *d* as healthcare providers with more narrow roles and focuses. Select nurses (option *a*) who have a broader role in interactions with clients.

3. Correct answer: d

Options *a, b,* and *d* are actions found in secondary prevention. Option *d,* health teaching, is mainly a focus in primary prevention.

Think of **p**rimary prevention as primary or first, where education of clients can **p**revent situations or illnesses. In **s**econdary prevention, **s**creening of clients occurs in an agency, in the home, or in an emergency.

4. Correct answer: a

Options *b, c,* and *d* can be subsumed under option *a,* since they are more specific and may be done as part of the action in option *a.*

The key words in the stem are "primary role," and the most global answer, option *a,* is most likely correct. The other options are too narrowly focused to be correct.

5. Correct answer: b

If the client is endangering self and others, the best approach is to use all available staff for the restraining. It does not matter if the staff are licensed or nonlicensed.

Be sure to read the question and responses carefully. This is not the time to use the rule of avoiding an option with an absolute. In this case, option *b* with "all," the absolute, is correct. Be cautious to avoid using rules without discretion.

▼ ▼ ▼ ▼ ▼ ▼ ▼ ▼ ▼ ▼   ▼ ▼ ▼

CHAPTER 5

Legal/Ethical Issues In Psychiatric Nursing

STUDY OUTCOMES

After completing this chapter, the reader will be able to do the following:

- ▼ Describe the commitment process.
- ▼ Identify civil and personal rights retained by psychiatric clients.
- ▼ Define the following terms: testamentary capacity, incompetency, confidentiality, and malpractice.
- ▼ Identify key issues related to client consent and to refusal of treatment.
- ▼ Discuss ethical issues in mental health psychiatric nursing.

KEY TERMS

Assault	Threat of touching someone without consent.
Battery	Unconsented touching.
Civil law	Relationships and disputes between citizens, usually involving a monetary settlement.
Civil rights	Constitutional rights.
Commitment	Legal procedure for hospitalization of clients against their will; usually relates to mental illness.
False imprisonment	Wrongful confinement of a person.
Malpractice	Civil action against a professional in which there is a failure to meet a professional standard, and the result is injury to the client.

CONTENT REVIEW

I. Hospital admission process (Table 5-1)

  A. Informal admission
1. Without formal or written application on client's part
2. Free to leave at any time
3. May leave "against medical advice" if they request a discharge

  B. Voluntary admission
1. Citizen of lawful age applies in writing
2. Agrees to receive treatment and abide by hospital rules
3. In most states, a parent or legal guardian can admit a child under age 16
4. Clients retain civil rights
    a. Right to vote
    b. Possess a driver's license
    c. Buy and sell property
    d. Manage personal affairs
    e. Hold office
    f. Practice a profession
    g. Engage in a business
5. May request a discharge
    a. Most states require a written notice
    b. Some states release immediately upon a request
    c. Some states detain for 48 hours to 15 days

  C. Involuntary admission: commitment
1. Legal criteria for commitment
    a. Dangerous to self

Table 5-1. Distinguishing Characteristics of the Three Types of Admission to Psychiatric Hospitals

Specific Factor	Informal Admission	Voluntary Admission	Involuntary Admission
Admission	No formal application needed	Formal application must be completed by patient	Application did not originate with patient
Discharge	Initiated by patient	Initiated by patient	Initiated by hospital or court but not by patient
Status of civil rights	Retained in full by patient	Retained in full by patient	Patient may retain some, none, or all, depending on state law
Justification	Voluntarily seeks help	Voluntarily seeks help	Mentally ill and one or more of the following ▼ Dangerous to others ▼ Dangerous to self ▼ Need for treatment

From Stuart G and Sundeen S, *Principles and practices of psychiatric nursing,* ed 4, St Louis, 1991, Mosby.

      b. Dangerous to others
      c. Need for treatment
  2. Process of commitment (Figure 5-1)
      a. Petition—by a relative, friend, public official, physician, interested party
      b. Examination—by one or two physicians; some states require one to be a psychiatrist
      c. Decision
        (1) Medical—a specified number of physicians
        (2) Court—formal hearing; client may request jury
        (3) Administrative—tribunal
        (4) Principle of "least restrictive alternative" (see "patient right" number 20)

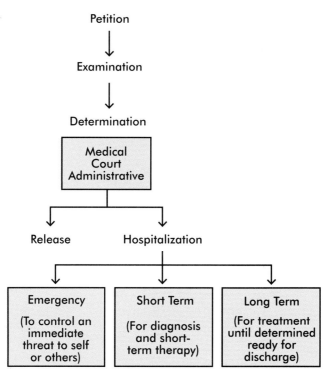

Figure 5-1. Diagram of the involuntary commitment process. (Modified from Stuart G and Sundeen S: *Principles and practice of psychiatric nursing,* ed 5, St Louis, 1995, Mosby.)

3. Types of commitment
   a. Emergency
      (1) Short-term
      (2) Immediate threat to self or others
      (3) Someone designated by the state files the petition
      (4) Report prepared by psychiatrist
      (5) Reviewed by judge or hospital official
      (6) Hospitalized 3 to 30 days
   b. Temporary hospitalization
      (1) Diagnosis established
      (2) Short-term therapy
      (3) Similar to emergency hospitalization
      (4) Time frame—2 to 6 months
      (5) Some states require a court order for temporary commitments
      (6) If client is not ready for discharge, petition can be filed for an indefinite commitment

      c. Indefinite hospitalization
- (1) Indefinite time
- (2) Usually court commitment
- (3) May consult a lawyer at any time to request a court hearing
- (4) Hospital may discharge client without going to court

4. Civil rights may or may not be retained, depending on the state

II. Client's rights

A. 1973 American Hospital Association issued the Patient's Bill of Rights

B. Clients presently have the following rights

1. Right to communicate with people outside the hospital through correspondence, telephone, and personal visits
- a. Visit and hold telephone conversations in privacy
- b. Send unopened letters to anyone
- c. Staff can limit access to telephone or visitors if harmful to the client
- d. Staff can limit times when calls are made and received and when visitors can enter the facility

2. Right to keep clothing and personal effects
- a. Valuable items left at home
- b. Staff can remove dangerous items

3. Right to be employed
- a. Payment for work therapy programs within the hospital
- b. Must be paid minimum wages

4. Right to religious freedom

5. Right to manage and dispose of property

6. Right to execute wills
- a. Testamentary capacity
- b. Must be able to
  - (1) Know he is making a will
  - (2) Know the nature and extent of the property
  - (3) Know who friends and relatives are
- c. Two or three people must witness the will

7. Right to enter into contractual relationships
- a. Incompetency
  - (1) Legal term
  - (2) Defect in judgment
  - (3) Incapability of handling own affairs
  - (4) Separate entity from commitment
  - (5) Client cannot marry, drive, or make contracts

8. Right to education
9. Right to habeas corpus—may request a hearing at any time to be released from the hospital
10. Right to make purchases
11. Right to an independent psychiatric examination
12. Right to retain licenses, privileges, or permits established by law, such as a driver's or professional license
13. Right to sue or be sued
14. Right to marry and divorce
15. Right not to be subject to unnecessary mechanical restraints
16. Right to privacy
    a. Professionals are responsible for protecting a client's right to confidentiality; *do not disclose that client is hospitalized*
    b. Privileged communication
       (1) Applies in court-related proceedings
       (2) Client can sue listener for disclosing information
       (3) Exists between clients and health professionals only if established by law—33 states recognize privileged communication
    c. Client records
       (1) Nurses' notes should be written carefully, since privileged communication does not apply
       (2) Charts can be brought into court
    d. Protecting a third party: health professional needs to break privileged communication in the threat of harm to others
17. Right to informed consent
    a. Physician should explain the treatment's possible complications and risks
    b. Client must be able to consent; not a minor or incompetent
    c. Failure to obtain may lead to assault and battery charges
18. Right to treatment
    a. Confinement without treatment is incarceration
    b. Team needs to show that treatment will improve or cure the client
    c. Individualized treatment plans are required
    d. Need to have qualified, sufficient number of staff
19. Right to refuse treatment; three criteria to treat over a client's objection
    a. Client behaviors exhibit a clear and present danger to self or others
    b. Treatment has a reasonable chance to benefit the client
    c. Client is incompetent to evaluate the necessity of treatment

20. Right to treatment in the least restrictive setting
    a. Outpatient versus inpatient
    b. Seclusion and restraints should be reserved for situations in which less restrictive means (medication, talking) have not worked and the situation of dangerousness is present
21. Right to accessible health care
22. Right to courteous and individualized health care
23. Right to information about the diagnosis, prognosis, and treatment
24. Right to information about the qualifications, names, and titles of personnel delivering care
25. Right to refuse observation by those not directly involved in care
26. Right to a coordination and continuity of health care
27. Right to information on the charges for services
    (Stuart G and Sundeen S, 1991)

III. Ethical considerations
A. Practitioners must identify right from wrong
B. Dilemmas exist when there is a possibility of good and harm in the same action
C. Dilemmas exist when there is a choice between two equally unsatisfactory alternatives
D. Ethical theories (Table 5-2)
    1. Libertarianism
        a. Individual is sovereign
        b. Free choice unless harmful to others

Table 5-2. Ethical Positions Toward a Psychiatric Client's Right to Refuse Treatment

Position	Attitude
Libertarian	The client may refuse any treatment if the client does not harm others
Paternalist	The mental health-psychiatric nurse may override a client's rights for the good of the client
Utilitarian	The mental health-psychiatric nurse may override a client's rights if doing so serves the greatest happiness of the greatest number
Rational paternalist	The client's rights may be overidden if the client would later regard such an action as being in the client's rational interest, and in contributing to his autonomy as a person

2. Paternalism
   a. One's father knows best
   b. Must comply with authority figures
   c. Position of power
3. Utilitarianism
   a. Greatest happiness for the greatest number
   b. Majority rule
4. Rational paternalist
   a. Client's rights may be overidden
   b. Client would later regard this as contribution to autonomy
5. Egoism
   a. One thinks and acts in one's own best interest
   b. Does not consider interests of others
6. Altruism—love, care, and consideration for the needs of others
7. Doctrine of double effect—lesser good or harm is permissible if done to achieve a greater good
8. Existentialism—human beings have free will and are responsible for their own acts

E. **Ethical/moral dilemmas confronting the nurse**
   1. Commitment
      a. Dangerousness is difficult to establish
         (1) What type of act is harmful?
         (2) What degree of injury constitutes harm?
         (3) How likely is it that the harmful act will occur?
      b. Ethical questions
         (1) Does freedom of choice include client's choice not to take medications?
         (2) Is coercion fair?
         (3) Could outpatient therapy be as effective?
         (4) What are the rights of the homeless people with mental illness?
         (5) What is appropriate housing for discharged clients?
   2. Restraints and seclusion
      a. What alternatives might be acceptable?
      b. Guideline for controlling behavior: always use the least restrictive means that are appropriate to the situation
      c. Have ongoing evaluation of the client
   3. Conflicts of interest generated by laws and theories
      a. Failing to medicate could deny the right to receive treatment
      b. Failing to medicate could cause the illness to continue

     c.   Failing to medicate could cause a psychosis, which could result in harm to self and others

     d.   Medicating without a clear threat of violence violates client's right to refuse treatment

4.   Nurses have legal obligations both to the agency and to clients. Nurses may be limited by institutional policies that circumscribe the nurses' authority to act.

5.   Nurses may work with physicians (usually considered to have the ultimate accountability for client care) whose behaviors suggests minimal or no respect for the client's rights

REVIEW QUESTIONS

1. Which behavior is inappropriate to have clients admitted in an involuntary manner?
    a. Danger to self
    b. Danger to others
    c. Hopelessness
    d. Threatening behavior

2. Determination of which individual behaviors are acceptable or unacceptable is most often made by
    a. Society
    b. Courts of law
    c. Psychiatric professionals
    d. Government regulations

3. If a client is given an injection after verbally refusing the medication, the nurse may be charged with
    a. Assault
    b. Malpractice
    c. Battery
    d. Negligence

4. Which one of these situations may be an example of false imprisonment?
    a. The client is confused and attempts to leave the facility. The nurse restrains the client and immediately obtains a physician's order.
    b. A psychotic client runs away from the unit. The staff chases the client and returns the client to the unit.
    c. A client has been bothersome all day. The staff places him in a seclusion room.
    d. An involuntary-admitted client leaves the hospital. The client is returned by hospital security.

5. A client states to the nurse, "I'm going to kill my wife when I get out of here." The nurse must
    a. Document this information after immediate notification of the physician
    b. Notify the client's wife immediately
    c. Contact the local law enforcement authorities
    d. Notify the hospital administration

ANSWERS, RATIONALES, AND TEST-TAKING TIPS

Rationales	Test-Taking Tips

1. **Correct answer: c**

   Hopelessness, although a characteristic and symptom of some mental health disorders, does not pose a threat to an individual or to others. The other options indicate a threat to others.

   The key words in the question are "behavior . . . inappropriate to treat . . . involuntary." Cluster options *a, b,* and *d* to associate that these indicate threats and may require involuntary admissions.

2. **Correct answer: a**

   Society establishes the norms by which its members will live. These norms will vary from society to society.

   If you have no idea of the correct answer, cluster options *b, c,* and *d* under the category of a specific group. Option *a,* society, being a more global category, is a best choice.

3. **Correct answer: c**

   Battery is defined as the touching of a person or anything else attached to a person without consent. Assault is the threat of touching someone without consent. Malpractice, a civil action against a health professional, is when there is a failure to meet a professional standard, with result of injury to the client. Negligence is the failure to act, with resultant harm to the client.

   Recall that all of these options, if enacted, would result in harm to the client. Associate assault with more auditory threats of harm. Associate battery with beating or with touching the body. Malpractice occurs from a nonstandard action; negligence is from nonstandard inaction.

4. **Correct answer: c**

   With false imprisonment there is lack of probable cause. In option *c* the action is an

   Eliminate options *a* and *b,* since in both the client has a dysfunction of mental thought. In option *d* the clue

inappropriate use (without just cause) of restraints or seclusion. The other options include just cause to retain the client.

to eliminate it is "involuntary admitted client." Option *c* describes no just cause for the seclusion.

5. Correct answer: a

The immediate step is to notify the physician. It is the physician who will give directions to notify the wife or authorities. All information must be documented on the client record as the client stated it.

The physician is the decision maker and leader in the client's care. The other options include those persons to contact after approval and the written orders from the physician.

Therapeutic Treatment Modalities

STUDY OUTCOMES

After completing this chapter, the reader will be able to do the following:

▼ Apply the nursing process to the various types of therapy:
individual
milieu
activity
group
family
somatic

▼ Describe the nursing care of clients receiving electroconvulsive, orthomolecular, or psychopharmacological treatments.

▼ Differentiate between functional and dysfunctional families.

▼ Identify for the four major classes of psychotropic drugs:
clinical indications
mode of action
pertinent side effects
client education needs
nursing implications

KEY TERMS

Alter egos	Persons who provide an additional interpretation of another person's verbalizations.
Boundaries	Rules that define who participates and how (Haber et al, 1992).
Catharsis	Outpouring of emotional tension through verbalization of feelings (Pasquali, 1989).
Crisis	Internal imbalance that results from a stressful event or perceived threat.
Electroconvulsive therapy (ECT)	Grand mal seizure is artificially induced by passing an electric current through electrodes applied to the temples.
External structure	Includes culture, neighbors, social class, status, environment, and extended family (Haber et al, 1992).
Family	Small social system made up of people held together by strong reciprocal affections and loyalties and living in a permanent household that persists over time (Haber et al, 1992).
Family composition	Defined by who lives in a specific household (Haber et al, 1992).
Fusion	Tendency of two or more people experiencing an intense emotional reaction to unite and lose personal boundaries.
Group	Collection of individuals with a common purpose.
Internal family structure	Family composition, rank order, subsystems, and boundaries (Haber et al, 1992).
Milieu	Use of the whole environment as a therapeutic agent.
Norms	Defined limits within which member behavior is considered acceptable.
Polypharmacy	Use of combinations of psychoactive drugs in a client at one time.
Psychodrama	Focus on dramatizing an individual's conflicts, problems, and relationships.
Psychosurgery (lobotomy)	Surgical intervention to sever fibers connecting one part of the brain with another, resulting in changed behavior, thought content, or mood.
Rank order	Position of a child in a family with respect to age (Haber et al, 1992).

Somatic therapy	Physiological approaches to treat clients with mental illness. It includes
	▼ Mechanical restraints
	▼ Seclusion or isolation
	▼ Psychosurgery
	▼ Electroconvulsive therapy
	▼ Orthomolecular therapy
	▼ Psychopharmacology
Therapeutic groups	Purpose is the personal and emotional growth of its members (Haber et al, 1992).

CONTENT REVIEW

TYPES OF THERAPEUTIC TREATMENT MODALITIES

▼ Individual
▼ Milieu
▼ Activity
▼ Group
▼ Family
▼ Somatic

INDIVIDUAL PSYCHOTHERAPY

I. Psychoanalytical treatment

A. Central concept—psychosexual issues

B. Involves the unconscious level of mental functioning

C. Disruptive behavior relates to earlier, unresolved developmental tasks

D. Symptoms are symbols of childhood conflicts. Example: washing hands to cleanse self from being labeled bad by Mom.

E. Elements of treatment

1. Free association—verbalize thoughts as they occur without censorship

2. Dream analysis

3. Transference

   a. Unconscious mechanism

   b. Feelings and attitudes associated with important people in one's early life are attributed to others in current relationships

4. Countertransference—conscious or unconscious emotional response by a staff member to a client

     5. PROS—elements for
       a. Clients recognize conflicts through therapist's interpretation of free association and dream analysis
       b. Therapist often represents earlier authority figure, which helps in resolving conflicts
     6. Cons—elements against
       a. Long-term process—several years
       b. Time-consuming
       c. Expensive
       d. Sexist

  F. **Roles of client and therapist**
     1. Client
       a. Active participant
       b. Reveals thoughts and dreams
       c. Lies down
         (1) Relaxes
         (2) Recreates childhood
     2. Therapist
       a. Impersonal
       b. Nonverbal clues not available due to positioning
       c. Verbal responses—noncommittal and brief
       d. Interprets behavior

  G. **Psychoanalytical therapists**
     1. Erik Erikson
     2. Anna Freud
     3. Sigmund Freud
     4. Melanie Klein
     5. Karen Hornay
     6. Frieda Fromm-Reichmann
     7. C.G. Jung

II. Interpersonal model

  A. **Central concept—behavior evolves around interpersonal relationships**
  B. **Also emphasizes early life experience**
  C. **Prominent theorists**
     1. Harry Stack Sullivan
     2. Hildegard Peplau
  D. **Anxiety associated with disapproval from significant others**
  E. **Therapeutic process**
     1. Corrective emotional experience
     2. Learn more satisfying interpersonal relationships through therapy

3. Unconditionally accepted by therapist
4. Relationship with therapist
   a. Builds trust
   b. Facilitates empathy
   c. Enhances self-esteem
5. Roles of client and therapist
   a. Therapist
      (1) Participant observer
      (2) Engages the client
      (3) Uncritical acceptance
   b. Client—shares concerns

III. Social model

A. Central concept—social conditions are responsible for maladaptive behavior
B. Thomas Szasz
   1. Myth of mental illness—believed no such thing as mental illness
   2. Believes society labels people who do not conform to culturally defined standards
   3. Thus he believes people are responsible for their behavior
   4. Objects to behavior's being labeled as mental illness
C. Therapeutic process
   1. Freedom of choice
   2. No involuntary hospitalization
   3. Focus on primary prevention
D. Roles of client and therapist
   1. Client
      a. Initiates therapy
      b. Defines problem
      c. Approves or rejects interventions
      d. Terminates when satisfied
   2. Therapist
      a. Collaborates
      b. Makes recommendations
      c. May be professionals or nonprofessionals with professional consultation

IV. Existential model

A. Central concept—experience in here and now
B. Major theorists
   1. Frederick Perls—gestalt therapy

      2. William Glasser—reality therapy

      3. Albert Ellis—rational-emotive therapy

C. Therapeutic process

      1. Returns client to awareness of his/her being. Example: going mad and regaining sanity.

      2. Focuses on encounter—appreciation by two individuals of the existence of each other

      3. Life is process of becoming

      4. Understand the past

      5. Live in present

      6. Look forward to future

      7. Rational-emotive therapy (Albert Ellis)

         a. Active

         b. Directive

         c. Cognitive

         d. Confrontive

         e. Assuming responsibility

         f. Self-acceptance

         g. Taking risks

      8. Reality therapy (William Glasser)

         a. Need for identity

         b. Recognition of life goals

         c. Impediments to accomplishing goals

         d. Oriented to present

         e. Focus on behavior not feelings

      9. Gestalt therapy (Frederick Perls)

         a. Here and now

         b. Identification of feelings

         c. Self-awareness

         d. Focus on body sensations

         e. Deal with unfinished business

D. Roles of client and therapist

      1. Therapist

         a. Acts as a guide to client

         b. Direct

         c. Caring

         d. Warm

         e. Open

         f. Honest

      2. Client

         a. Accepts responsibility

         b. Dependence discouraged

  c. Treated as adult
  d. Illness deemphasized
  e. Active participant

V. Behavior model
 A. **Central concept—focus is on client's behavior**
 B. **Theorists**
  1. B.F. Skinner
  2. Joseph Wolpe
 C. **Therapeutic process**
  1. Stimulus presented—behavior occurs—behavior reinforced
  2. Emphasis on effect of environment on human behavior
  3. Behavior must be described
  4. Positive and negative reinforcement both increase chances of behavior's recurring
  5. Aversion therapy
   a. Painful stimulus, usually electric shock to create aversion to stimulus
   b. Moral-ethical conflicts related to this treatment of client
   c. Client must agree
   d. Emotional pain outweighs physical pain
  6. Token economy
   a. Encourages socially acceptable behavior
   b. Tokens given for desirable behaviors
   c. Tokens turned in for snacks, passes
   d. Action reinforces future repetition of desired behavior
   e. Points may be substituted for tokens
   f. Reward needs to be of value to the client
 D. **Roles of client and therapist**
  1. Therapist
   a. Teacher
   b. Behavioral expert
   c. Helps client unlearn and replace symptoms
   d. Establishes behavioral objectives
   e. No exploration of client's past
   f. No insight oriented therapy
  2. Client
   a. Active participant
   b. Homework assignments
   c. Student role

VI. Medical model

A. Central concept—traditional psychiatrist-client relationship

B. Based on diagnosis of mental illness

C. Somatic treatments

    1. Pharmacology

    2. Electroconvulsive therapy

D. Physician is leader of team

E. Elements of other models may also be used simultaneously

F. Functions of model

    1. Treat the illness

    2. Avoid placing blame for behavior

    3. Focus on healing instead of blaming (Stuart and Sundeen, 1995)

G. Illness relates to disorder of the central nervous system synaptic levels of neurotransmitters

    1. Dopamine

    2. Serotonin

    3. Norepinephrine

H. Environmental and social factors may

    1. Predispose to illness

    2. Precipitate the illness

I. Therapeutic process

    1. Physician examination

        a. Psychosocial assessment

        b. Physical assessment

    2. Diagnosis according to *Diagnostic and Statistical Manual of Mental Disorders,* ed 4 (DSM IV)

    3. Treatment

        a. Pharmacology

        b. Electroconvulsive therapy

        c. Short-term psychotherapy

        d. Treatment over when client subjectively feels better

J. Roles of client and therapist

    1. Physician

        a. Healer

        b. Institutes treatment plan

    2. Client

        a. Admits illness

        b. Complies with treatment

VII. Nursing model—central concepts

A. Holistic approach

    1. Biological

      2. Psychological
      3. Sociocultural
  B. Collaborative effort between nurse and client
  C. Observe and interpret behaviors
  D. Concerned with emotional response to problems
  E. Nurse acts as client advocate
  F. Nurse theorists
      1. Ida Jean Orlando
      2. Hildegard Peplau
      3. Imogene King
      4. Dorothea Orem
      5. Joan Riehl
      6. Sister Callista Roy
      7. Martha Rogers
  G. Focus is on client responses to a risk for or actual health problems
  H. Nursing diagnoses focus on behaviors
  I. Care of clients based on the nursing process
  J. Nurse-client relationship based on mutuality

VIII. Crisis intervention

  A. Crisis (Figure 6-1)—central concepts
      1. External stressful event leads to imbalance
      2. Old coping skills are ineffective
      3. Anxiety and tension increase
      4. Disorganized behavior results
      5. Time limited—1 to 6 weeks
  B. Causes of crisis
      1. Loss
      2. Transition
         a. Mourning
         b. Graduation
         c. Marriage
         d. Birth of a child
      3. Several events occurring simultaneously—cluster of events
  C. Four phases of a crisis
      1. Phase 1—external precipitating event(s)
      2. Phase 2
         a. Perception of threat
         b. Anxiety increases
         c. May cope and resolve crisis

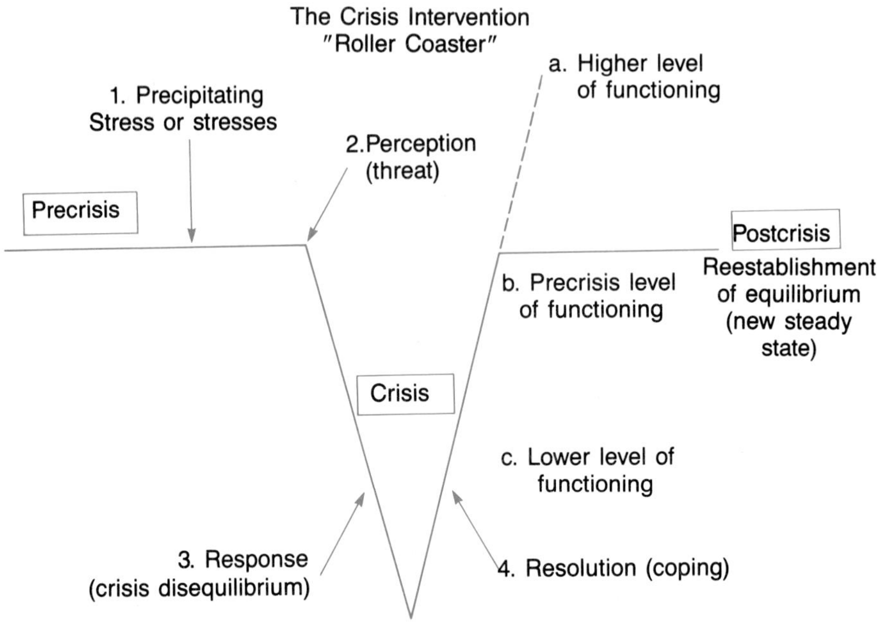

Figure 6-1. Crisis intervention roller coaster. (From Haber J et al: *Comprehensive psychiatric nursing,* ed 4, St Louis, 1992, Mosby.)

3. Phase 3
   a. Failure of coping
   b. Increasing disorganization
   c. Physical symptoms
      (1) Racing thoughts
      (2) Disturbed concentration
      (3) Eating disorders
      (4) Sleeping disorders
      (5) Relationship problems
4. Phase 4
   a. Mobilization of internal and external resources
   b. Three possible resolutions related to pre-crisis functioning
      (1) Higher level of functioning
      (2) Same level of functioning
      (3) Lower level of functioning
D. **Balancing factors for a crisis**
   1. Realistic perception of event
   2. Situational supports
   3. Adequate coping mechanisms

E. **Types of crises**
 1. Maturational characteristics
    a. Predictable life events
    b. Role transitions
    c. Onset gradual
    d. Resolutions gradual
    e. May inhibit progression to future developmental stages
    f. Example: retirement, job change, marriage, parenthood
 2. Situational characteristics
    a. Unanticipated events
    b. Disequilibrium
    c. Unpreparedness for event
    d. Examples: change in financial status; loss of work from injuries, divorce, death of a friend
 3. Social characteristics
    a. Accidental, unanticipated
    b. Uncommon
    c. Involve multiple losses, environmental changes
    d. Example: natural disaster, civil riot, violent crime
F. **Crisis intervention—application of the nursing process**
 1. Assessment
    a. Collect data
    b. Establish rapport
    c. Assess three areas
       (1) Perception of precipitating event by client
       (2) Client's strengths and weaknesses
       (3) Nature and strength of situational supports
    d. Event has usually occurred within 10 to 14 days of client's seeking help
    e. Examples of questions to ask
       (1) Why did you come for help today?
       (2) What happened in your life that is different?
       (3) How does this problem affect your life today?
       (4) How have you handled other crises in your life?
       (5) Is there someone with whom you are particularly close?
       (6) Are you involved in any community activities?
 2. Planning
    a. Analyzed assessment data
    b. Compare past and present events and responses
    c. Explore alternative solutions
    d. Explore specific interventions

3. Intervention
   a. Is goal directed
   b. Connections made between meaning of event and crisis
   c. Feelings of client acknowledged
   d. Provide opportunities for expression and validation of feelings
   e. Explore alternative coping skills
   f. Client tries out new behaviors
   g. Therapist is directive
4. Evaluation
   a. Compare goals with behavioral outcome
   b. Consolidate learning
   c. May refer to additional therapy for unresolved issues

MILIEU THERAPY

I. Overview
A. Definition—the environment is designed to facilitate rehabilitation
B. Nurses have greatest responsibility for maintaining the environment
   1. Twenty-four hours per day
   2. Seven days per week
C. Authority and accountability shared by team members
D. Treatment modalities
   1. Art
   2. Music
   3. Poetry
   4. Movement therapy
   5. Psychodrama
   6. Individual therapy
   7. Family therapy
   8. Group therapy
   9. Client governance

II. Historical development
A. Maxwell Jones—use of whole environment as the therapeutic agent
   1. Whole environment is a protective setting
   2. Factors that foster a healthy personality
      a. Therapeutic interventions
      b. Physical environment
      c. Interpersonal relationships

     3. Environment viewed as a microcosm of society
     4. Focus is to explore interactions with others in environment
     5. Behaviors of hostility, manipulation, insensitivity, lack of responsibility, and poor judgement are confronted by entire community

III. Principles of therapeutic community (milieu)

A. Responsibility for treatment belongs to the staff and the client
B. Roles of staff and clients are equalized—may discuss either staff behavior or client behavior
C. Democratic environment is fostered
D. Open communication is encouraged
E. Focus is on clients' assets
F. Interpersonal interactions are utilized to improve communication skills
G. Autonomy is reinforced
H. Individuals are held responsible for own actions
I. Peer pressure is utilized to reinforce rules and regulations
J. Inappropriate behaviors are dealt with as they occur
K. Group discussion and temporary seclusion are favored approaches for acting-out behavior
L. Team approach is used
M. Clients are treated as part of team and share in the responsibility and process of making decisions
N. Clients are involved in all phases of treatment
O. Community government is set up
     1. Use meetings to teach standards, values, and behavior
     2. Explore behaviors
     3. Try new roles
     4. Make decisions
     5. Use problem solving (Pasquali, 1989)
P. Two main goals for clients
     1. Learn to set limits
     2. Learn psychosocial skills

IV. Psychosocial skills development

A. Leadership—client government (may serve as officer or committee chairperson)
B. Self-assertion
     1. Expressing feelings and attitudes is encouraged in milieu
     2. Focus is on "talking it out"

C. Occupational activities
   1. Basic skills for managing life
   2. Activities of daily living
   3. Vocational counseling, training
D. Recreational activities
   1. Leisure activities
   2. Cooperation with others
   3. Conversation within social context
E. Independence
   1. Focus on decision making
   2. Problem solving
   3. Self-care

V. Setting limits within milieu
A. Setting limits provides safety
B. Behaviors that require setting limits
   1. Destructive
      a. Suicide
      b. Homicide
      c. Harm to persons or property
   2. Disorganized
      a. Psychotic behaviors
         (1) Hallucinations
         (2) Delusions
         (3) Disoriented
      b. Dissociative episodes of posttraumatic stress disorder
   3. Deviant
      a. Acting out
      b. Breaking rules
      c. Illegal activities
   4. Dysphoric
      a. Depressed
      b. Withdrawn
      c. Elated
      d. Phobic
      e. Obsessive-compulsive
   5. Dependent—avoids responsibility for thoughts and behaviors

VI. Physical structure of milieu
A. Homelike atmosphere
B. Nursing station open and accessible
C. Street clothes for clients and staff

D. Breakproof glass versus barred windows
E. Day rooms resembling living rooms
F. Dining room
G. Recreation rooms
H. Tranquil colors

VII. Programs within milieu
A. Client government
   1. Structured meeting
   2. Clients and staff
   3. Clients have input into all unit activities
   4. May make decisions related to privileges for other clients
   5. Discussion of unit problems of everyday living
   6. Usually meet once per week
B. Work-related activities
   1. Work therapy
   2. Monetary reward
   3. Client should choose type of work
   4. Work geared toward job-related skills
   5. Offer a variety of activities (Rawlins et al, 1993)

VIII. Role of the nurse in milieu therapy
A. Assessing and intervening in medical problems
B. Distributing medication
C. Planning programs
D. Coordinating team activities
E. Managing the milieu
F. Working with clients individually
G. Leading groups
H. Participating in community meetings
I. Coordinating medical care
J. Administering medications
K. Working with families

IX. Pros and cons of milieu therapy
A. Pros
   1. Each client owns own behavior
   2. Peer pressure is useful and powerful
   3. Client's environment is part of treatment
   4. Every interaction is opportunity for therapeutic intervention
   5. Inappropriate behaviors are dealt with as they occur
   6. Restriction and punishment avoided

      7. Self-esteem built through ownership process

      8. Mimics outside environment

B. Cons

      1. Staff needs to be comfortable with equality with clients

      2. Conflict resolution is needed as part of the staff's skills

      3. Low client-to-staff ratio

      4. Requires continuous open communication among all staff and clients

ACTIVITY THERAPY

I. Common types of activity therapy

A. Poetry therapy

      1. Purposes

          a. Alter mood. Example: depressed client reads a sad poem with line of hope.

          b. Explore feelings

          c. Increase self-esteem

          d. Increase ego strength

          e. Decrease duration and intensity of anxiety

          f. Decrease isolation

          g. Increase emotional insight

          h. Promote identification with other clients who have similar conflicts, anxieties, and feelings

      2. Process

          a. Leader selects poem to be read in a group and then poem is discussed among group members; poem addresses problems, feelings, and lifestyles of group members

          b. Leader presents several poems with different themes; group picks poem for discussion

          c. Members write own poetry

B. Psychodrama

      1. Developed by Dr. Jacob Moreno

      2. Purposes for clients to

          a. Dramatize conflicts, problems, past and present relationships

          b. Increase insight related to conflicts, problems, and relationships

          c. Learn new ways to respond to conflicts, problems, and relationships

      3. Process

          a. Therapist directs scene

      b. Clients and/or staff members play key roles or act as alter egos (persons who provide an additional interpretation of another person's verbalizations)

      c. Role reversals are used to provide insights into the perceptions of others

      d. Catharsis of feelings promoted

      e. Therapist protects and interprets

      f. Reduces anxiety at end through a sharing session when group discusses relevant topics

    4. Use cautiously with schizophrenics

      a. They may have increased psychotic symptoms

      b. They may confuse "process" with "reality"

      c. They may be overwhelmed by unconscious material

C. Art therapy

    1. Purposes

      a. Provides pictorial overview of life

        (1) Feelings of loss

        (2) Separation

        (3) Disconnection

        (4) Love

        (5) Joy

      b. Stimulates self-expression, particularly in clients not in touch with feelings, such as schizophrenics

      c. Increases self-esteem

      d. Externalizes conflicts

      e. Provides safer means of communication for those lacking in trust

      f. Encourages analytical interpretation of conflicts

      g. Increases interpersonal interaction

    2. Process

      a. Leader gives theme to group and asks for responses

      b. Artistic ability is not a requisite

      c. Group could create collage—cooperation and interaction is encouraged

D. Movement therapy

    1. Purposes

      a. Promotes interpersonal interaction

      b. Increases physical well-being

      c. Increases self-esteem

      d. Reduces anxiety

      e. Provides outlet for fun

       2. Types
         a. Dance
         b. Exercise
         c. Yoga
  E. **Music therapy**
     1. Purposes
       a. Increases self-esteem through achievement
       b. Increases interpersonal interaction
       c. Increases attention span
       d. Has a calming effect
       e. Facilitates communication of feelings
       f. Provides leisure activity
       g. Promotes reminiscing
     2. Process
       a. Individual writes song
       b. Individual learns to play an instrument
       c. Individual performs solo
       d. Group writes song
       e. Group listens
       f. Group sings and performs
  F. **Journaling**
     1. Purposes
       a. Allows self-expression
       b. Provides catharsis of feelings
       c. Increases insight
       d. Increases awareness of feelings
     2. Process
       a. Unstructured—recording of impressions, feelings, and events as they occur
       b. Structured—exercise given by group leader. Example: "Write about a happy event in your life."
       c. Discussion of writing with others

II. Role of the nurse

  A. Nurses are not art, occupational, or recreational therapists
  B. Encourage client participation and validate recognition of therapeutic value
  C. Suggest activities to other therapists from knowledge of clients' interests
  D. Observe and report clients' responses to activities
  E. Plan and participate in activities

GROUP THERAPY

I. Structure of group therapy

A. Purpose—treatment modality

B. Four major goals
1. Decrease anxiety
2. Alleviate stress
3. Improve interpersonal relationships
4. Test out new behaviors

C. Inpatient settings
1. Open membership—constantly adding or losing members
2. Meet three to five times per week
3. Short-term

D. Outpatient settings
1. Longer duration
2. Meet once per week
3. Closed membership—do not add members

E. Group size
1. 7 to 10 members
2. If too few, not enough sharing
3. If too large, some feel excluded

F. Group length
1. 45 to 60 minutes—lower functioning
2. 90 to 120 minutes—higher functioning

G. Leader responsibility
1. Analyzes communication patterns
   a. Seating arrangements
   b. Common themes
   c. Who talks to whom
   d. Individual member communication
   e. How frequently the members speak
   f. How the group handles silence
   g. What topics the group avoids
2. Supplies feedback about communication process—individual and group
3. Structures the group according to time, place, procedures
4. Establishes structural rules
   a. Confidentiality
   b. Contacts outside of group
5. Accepts all members unconditionally
6. Encourages open expression of feelings
7. Encourages all members to verbally participate

      8. Intervenes to keep anxiety level within acceptable limits
      9. Accepts group in the here and now and its level of functioning
    10. Controls boundaries
        a. Starts and ends on time
        b. Prevents nongroup members from entering
        c. Intervenes to protect group members from direct interrogation

H. Group norms
    1. Are the rules of the group
    2. Define the limits for the group
    3. Act as a guide
    4. Examples (Box 6-1)
    5. May be
      a. Explicit—stated
      b. Implicit—implied
    6. Are necessary to reach goals

I. Group roles (Table 6-1)
    1. Maintain group
    2. Contribute to group tasks
    3. Contribute to individual goals
    4. Roles may change throughout group meetings
    5. Each member has a role

J. Group process—how things are discussed
    1. Everything that happens during the group
    2. Underlying dynamics
    3. Conflicts

Box 6-1. Group Rules

Attendance is expected at all group meetings.
Prompt arrival at each group meeting is expected.
Participation in/or attention to the group interaction is expected.
All feelings are valid and are not to be criticized.
Only one person speaks at a time.
No smoking or eating during group meeting.
Physically aggressive behavior is not allowed; no hitting or throwing of objects is permitted.
Leaving during a group meeting will mean not being able to return during that session.
What is discussed in group meeting remains in the group.
Group members are expected to work together to achieve group goals.

Haber J, et al: *Comprehensive psychiatric nursing*, ed 4, St Louis, 1992, Mosby.

Table 6-1. Group Member Roles According to Function

Group Maintenance	Group Task	Individual Goals
Encourager—praises others; agrees with and accepts the ideas of others; open to differences within the group *Harmonizer*—mediates and reconciles intragroup differences *Compromiser*—operates to resolve conflicts; seeks a compromise that all can accept	*Initiator*—offers new ideas, suggests solutions *Elaborator*—gives examples, develops meanings and explanations *Evaluator*—relates the group standards to any problem *Coordinator*—clarifies relationships among ideas and activities of the group	*Aggressor*—acts negatively with hostility toward others; jokes aggressively; attacks the group and its members *Recognition Seeker*—calls attention to own activities; boasts about achievements; redirects conversation toward self *Help Seeker or Confessor*—uses group to express nongroup-oriented feelings and thoughts; uses group to gain sympathy; expresses insecurity and self-deprecation *Dominator*—asserts authority and manipulates individuals and the group as a whole

Pasquali E, Arnold H, DeBasio N: *Mental health nursing: A holistic approach,* ed 3, St Louis, 1989, Mosby.

    4. Interpersonal relationships
    5. Atmosphere
    6. Norms
    7. Cohesiveness
  K. Group content—what is discussed
  L. Cohesiveness—characteristics of members
    1. Open to change
    2. Supportive of each other
    3. Internalize norms
    4. Focus on tasks

      5. Mutual bonds
      6. Common purpose
      7. Cooperation
      8. Committed to group
      9. Punctual to meetings
    10. Willing to take risks
    11. Mutual respect
    12. Open, honest exchange

M. Setting
    1. Adequate number of chairs
    2. Chairs arranged in a circle
    3. Eliminate barriers—no table
    4. Privacy essential—no open doors during group
    5. Accessibility to bathroom
    6. Adequate ventilation
    7. Comfortable temperature

II. Four stages of group development

A. Pregroup: forming of the group
    1. Time period before people know each other in the group setting
    2. Tasks to be completed
      a. Selecting group members
      b. Deciding the length and frequency of meetings
      c. Deciding composition of group membership
        (1) Homogeneous—members share common characteristics such as age, problem
        (2) Heterogenous—vary in characteristics
    3. Leader responsibilities
      a. Establishes purpose
      b. Secures physical space
      c. Selects members
      d. Decides if group to have closed or open status
      e. Screens interviewees
        (1) Determines member motivation
        (2) Describes norms
        (3) Educates about group
        (4) Determines compatibility of goals
        (5) Secures commitment to group
        (6) Begins leader/member relationship

B. Initial stage
    1. Group members have anxiety about being accepted

2. Tasks
    a. Setting of norms
    b. Casting of roles
3. Orientation period
    a. Member behaviors
        (1) Determining level of participation
        (2) Concerned with acceptance
        (3) Fear of rejection
        (4) Fear of self-disclosure
        (5) Fear that individual goals will not match group goals
        (6) Dependent on leader
        (7) Look to leader for structure, approval, acceptance
    b. Leader behaviors
        (1) Directive
        (2) Active
        (3) Group contract development
            (a) Goals
            (b) Confidentiality
            (c) Meeting times
            (d) Honesty expected
            (e) Structure
            (f) Rules
        (4) Encourages interaction between members
        (5) Facilitates approach/avoidance—to disclose too
            much information too early is discouraged
        (6) Suggests how group members might be helpful to
            one another
4. Conflict stage within initial stage
    a. Member behaviors
        (1) Focus on issues of control, power, authority
        (2) Members concerned with status in group
        (3) Dependency conflict
        (4) Struggle between independent and dependent issues
        (5) Independent members—attempt to take leader's role
        (6) Dependent members—ask leader for more direction
        (7) Subgroups form
        (8) Hostility toward leader or other members
    b. Leader behaviors
        (1) Allows expression of negative and positive feelings
        (2) Helps group understand conflict
        (3) Prevents scapegoating
        (4) Encourages direct expression of hostility

      c. Outcome
          (1) Leader is humanized
          (2) Responsibility for group is shared
          (3) Anger does not destroy leader
          (4) Conflict increases group's productivity
   5. Cohesive stage within initial stage
      a. Member behaviors
          (1) Form attachment to group
          (2) Positive feelings toward group and members
          (3) Self-disclosure
          (4) Suppress hostility
          (5) Limited problem solving
      b. Leader behaviors
          (1) Encourages problem solving
          (2) Demonstrates that differing opinions are acceptable
      c. Outcome: members accept that
          (1) Differences are okay
          (2) Differences help group to grow
          (3) Group can be productive

C. **Working stage**
   1. Group becomes team
   2. Group completes tasks
   3. Group shares responsibility
   4. Anxiety is decreased
   5. Group is stable
   6. Member behaviors
      a. Serious work occurs
      b. Explore goals and tasks
      c. Explore feelings
      d. Explore new coping mechanisms
   7. Leader behaviors
      a. Decreases activity
      b. Serves as consultant
      c. Keeps group on track
      d. Fosters cohesion
      e. Maintains boundaries
      f. Encourages work on tasks
      g. Helps group solve problems
   8. Outcome
      a. Group begins to achieve goals
      b. The need for the group decreases
      c. Sense of accomplishment among members

D. Termination stage
   1. Two types
      a. Whole group ends
      b. Individual member leaves
   2. Involves grieving and sense of loss
   3. Member behaviors
      a. Anger
      b. Regression
         (1) Dependency
         (2) Competition
      c. Avoidance
         (1) Do not come to group
         (2) Do not talk about termination
      d. May discuss other endings
         (1) Separations
         (2) Death
         (3) Aging
      e. Devalue group
      f. Sense of resolution
   4. Leader behaviors
      a. Reminisces about group's activities
      b. Evaluates group goals
      c. Discusses contributions of individual group members
      d. Encourages full discussion of termination for several
         sessions
      e. Shares own experience and feelings related to the group
      f. Discourages premature termination of individual group
         members

III. Support groups
A. General problem support groups
   1. Increase members' social network
   2. Members share common problems and solutions
   3. Members alter perceptions of selves and others
   4. Members realize they are not alone in experiences
   5. Usually led by nonprofessionals who experience the same
      problem
   6. Examples
      a. Alcoholics Anonymous
      b. Narcotics Anonymous
      c. Overeaters Anonymous
      d. Women's groups
      e. Men's groups

B. Medical problem support groups—for clients with medical problems
1. Usually professionally led
2. Support to clients with medical problems
3. Examples of common problems
   a. Brain injury
   b. Diabetes
   c. Mental illness
   d. Arthritis
C. Caregiver support groups
1. Professionally led
2. Support to family members of acutely or chronically ill
3. Examples of common groups
   a. Alzheimer's disease
   b. Children with leukemia
   c. Older adults
4. Goals of caregiver group members
   a. Increase coping skills
   b. Socialization
   c. Connection with community support services
   d. Maintenance of caregiver's health
5. Leader behaviors
   a. Educates
   b. Supports
   c. Encourages ventilation of feelings
6. Member concerns
   a. Finances
   b. Restriction of freedom
   c. Feelings of anger and loss
   d. Anonymity
D. Bereavement groups—goals for members
1. Support to grieving individuals
2. Outlet for expression of grief and loss
3. Managing loneliness
4. Socialization
5. Adapting to a new lifestyle

FAMILY INTERVENTIONS

I. Functional families
A. Flexible
B. Adapt to change

    C. Fusion is avoided

    D. Twosomes solve problems without involving a third person

    E. Differences encouraged

    F. All members assume responsibility for own behaviors

    G. Clear communication

    H. Clear generational boundaries

    I. Emotional distress in one member is viewed as function partially of all members—awareness of own boundaries and feelings remains

II. Dysfunctional families

    A. Members are self-centered

    B. Boundaries are rigid—minimal outside contacts

    C. Family perceived as chaotic

    D. Authority is inconsistent or lacking

    E. Roles are fused—unclear who is parent or child

    F. Individualism is discouraged

    G. Conflict is perceived as negative

    H. Communication is cold and distant

    I. No common goals identified

III. Family systems theory

    A. Developed by Murray Bowen

    B. Fluid, ever-changing system

    C. Change in one part of system necessitates changes in other parts

    D. Understood only as a whole

    E. Symptoms in one family member are evidence of dysfunction in family

    F. Goal of therapy: distinguish between thinking and feeling processes

    G. Families with fusion of thinking and feeling function poorly

    H. Differentiation of self

        1. Undifferentiated

            a. Family members know each other's thoughts and feelings

            b. Rigid

            c. Not adaptable

            d. Emotionally dependent

            e. Emotional oneness

        2. Differentiated

            a. Separation between thought and emotion

            b. Flexible

        c. Adaptable

        d. Emotionally interdependent

I. **Triangles**
1. Three-sided emotional connection in families
2. Emotional process occurs when a relationship is in difficulty
3. Composition
   a. Three people
   b. Two people and a group. Example: Alanon, a support group for the family members of alcoholics
   c. Two people and an issue. Example: drinking.
   d. Two people and an object. Example: house.
4. Difficult to have closeness without fusion
5. Triangles promote distance
6. Stabilize by avoiding tension, conflict, or painful issues
7. Not static; change with stress

J. **Multigenerational transmission**
1. Patterns of communication passed from generation to generation
2. Family norms, behaviors, problems, and patterns of relationships passed from generation to generation

K. **Family projection process**
1. Process through which differentiation problems of parents are transmitted to one or more children
2. Child becomes scapegoat
3. Child acts out his or her conflicts

L. **Subsystems**
1. Subgroups within family system
2. Usually three subsystems
   a. Marital
   b. Parental
   c. Sibling

M. **Boundaries**
1. Separateness of system, subsystem, or individual from environment
2. Clear boundaries necessary for functional families
3. Enmeshment = diffuse boundaries
4. Disengaged = extreme separateness
5. Families vacillate according to family stress

N. **Three family patterns**
1. Rigidity
   a. No change
   b. No conflict
   c. Public image of normalcy

      2. Overprotectiveness
        a. Members hypersensitive to emotional stress in other family members
        b. Nurturing behavior
        c. Decreased autonomy
        d. Decreased sense of competence—cannot do things
      3. Conflict avoidance
        a. Keep peace at any cost
        b. Issues remain unresolved and recycle

O. **Three pathological communication patterns**
      1. Disqualification
        a. Contradictions
        b. Inconsistencies
      2. Disconfirmation (invalidating)—"You don't really feel that way."
      3. Double bind
        a. Two simultaneous conflicting messages
        b. No-win situation
        c. Either response is inappropriate
        d. "Damned if you do, damned if you don't"

P. **Pseudomutuality**
      1. Rigid style of relating
      2. Common findings
        a. Confusion
        b. Distance
        c. Hostility
      3. False mutuality present—family members appear close

IV. Application of the nursing process with families

A. **Assessment**
      1. Structure
        a. Boundaries
        b. Subsystems
        c. Culture
      2. Developmental stage
        a. Marriages
        b. Ages of children and grandchildren
        c. Patterns of behavior
        d. Attachments
      3. Functioning
        a. Work in household
        b. Daily routines
        c. Communication patterns

    4. Goals of assessment
       a. Trace history of family
       b. Discover how symptoms developed
       c. Assess reactions to illness in family
    5. Genogram
       a. Illustration of family structures over three generations
       b. Assessment tool to look at family function
       c. Usually gathered from all family members but may just be client
       d. Focus first on the presenting problem of the client
       e. Move to system attitude. Example: "The information I am asking for will help me understand how your problem developed."
       f. Information needed
          (1) Names
          (2) Ages
          (3) Dates
             (a) Deaths
             (b) Births
             (c) Marriages
             (d) Separations
             (e) Divorces
             (f) Moves
             (g) Illness—physical or mental illness of family members
          (4) Physical location of family members
          (5) Frequency of contact between family members
          (6) Sibling position
          (7) Characteristics of relationships
       g. Ecomap
          (1) Overview of nuclear family as it relates to neighborhood and community
          (2) External family structure

B. Possible family diagnoses
    1. Ineffective family coping
    2. Disorder of sexual boundaries
    3. Marital conflict
    4. Risk for physical abuse
    5. Codependency

C. Outcome criteria
    1. Goals established by family
       a. Anxiety related to client will decrease

      b. Family will motivate client to increase activity

      c. Family locates community resources

      d. Members know essential information about medications

      e. Family gains control over household

      f. Members accept illness of family member

      g. Members exhibit increased individuation

D. General nursing interventions

  1. Act as a family advocate

  2. Communicate with other health team members

  3. Educate family about medications

  4. Facilitate involvement with community support services

  5. Remain differentiated from family

E. Specific nursing interventions

  1. Enmeshed (fused) families

      a. Identify most individuated member and encourage him/her to be more separate. Example: engage in social relationships outside the family.

      b. Encourage family to make "I" statements

      c. Encourage realignment of responsibilities among family members

  2. Family violence

      a. Set limits on acting-out behavior

      b. Refer family to community resources that treat victims of family violence

      c. Help family identify available supports

      d. Assess family members for evidence of abuse

      e. Help family meet needs of dependent family members, such as older adults, physically ill, children

  3. Codependent behaviors

      a. Characteristics

         (1) Invested in controlling others

         (2) Responsible for meeting others' needs instead of own

         (3) Enmeshment in relationships

         (4) Constricted emotions

         (5) Rigid or diffuse boundaries

      b. Nursing interventions with codependent behaviors

         (1) Encourage self-help groups. Example: Adult Children of Alcoholics (ACOA).

         (2) Encourage assertiveness training

         (3) Encourage marital counseling

SOMATIC THERAPY

I. Two approaches to physical restraints

   A. Mechanical restraints

      1. Require physician's order

      2. Types

         a. Camisoles or canvas jackets

         b. Padded leather, plastic, cloth

            (1) Wrist

            (2) Ankle

            (3) Waist

         c. Sheet restraints or canvas bedsheets fastened to bed frame

      3. Reasons for use

         a. Risk of injury to self

         b. Unresponsiveness to sedative or antipsychotic medication

         c. Confusion—results in wandering off or falls

         d. Need for rest

         e. Need for decreased stimuli

         f. Client's request for sense of safety or control

         g. Client is potentially harmful to others

      4. *Should be utilized as last resort after less restrictive interventions have proved ineffective*

      5. Applying restraints

         a. Give support and reassurance

         b. Explain use

         c. Have adequate personnel—licensed and unlicensed

         d. Nurse assigns staff duties for application

            (1) Securing arms

            (2) Securing legs

            (3) Talking to client

            (4) Clearing the area

            (5) Talking to other clients

      6. Nursing interventions

         a. Check vital signs according to policy

         b. Bathe and provide skin care

         c. Take to bathroom or provide bedpan or urinal—frequency per agency protocol

         d. Position extremities correctly, anatomically

         e. Pad restraints

         f. Offer food and fluids per agency protocol

    g. Release each limb in rotation according to agency policy to maintain circulation and prevent nerve damage

    h. Do not leave alone—observe constantly or arrange for someone to be in the room

  7. Camisole restraints

    a. Canvas jacket with arms tied across the body

    b. Prevents client from striking out

  8. Sheet restraints

    a. Hole in sheet for client's head

    b. Often used with wrist and ankle restraints

    c. Requires continuous nursing observation

    d. Used only for extreme agitation and for short periods

B. Seclusion or isolation

  1. Client is confined alone in a single room

  2. Locked or unlocked room

  3. Mattress on floor, no bed (safety precaution)

  4. Purposes of seclusion

    a. Containment—prevent harm to self or others

    b. Isolation—has a decreased need to relate to others

    c. Decreased sensory input

  5. Contraindications

    a. Medical instability

    b. Risk for self-harm

    c. Very warm room

  6. Procedure

    a. Designate leader

    b. Have enough staff

    c. Clear the area

    d. Communicate clearly with client

    e. Move client—may require restraining or client may move voluntarily

    f. Remove clothing and dangerous objects

    g. Debrief staff after incident

  7. Nursing interventions

    a. Provide food and fluids

    b. Encourage use of bathroom

    c. Observe frequently

    d. Observe through window if possible

    e. Assess regularly for continued needs

    f. Communicate with client as needed

II. Psychosurgery: surgical intervention to sever fibers connecting one part of the brain with another, resulting in changed behavior, thought content, or mood. Example: lobotomy.

A. Used with chronic depression and obsessional conditions with high anxiety

B. Used only as last resort and very infrequently

C. Current techniques utilize lasers

D. Permanent and irreversible

E. Current techniques minimize damage to personality and social functioning

F. Client must sign consent form

G. Nursing care concerns
   1. Major effect is emotional not intellectual
   2. Client's hallucinations may continue
   3. 60% of clients improve significantly
   4. This surgery raises major moral and ethical issues related to control of behavior and emotional responses

H. Pros
   1. Decreased anxiety
   2. Decreased obsessive thoughts
   3. Decreased depressed mood

I. Cons
   1. Flattened affect
   2. Decreased emotional response

III. Electroconvulsive Therapy

A. Action of ECT—theory
   1. Electric current and seizure activity in brain produce changes in neurotransmitters and receptor sites
   2. Grand mal seizure is artifically induced by passing an electric current through electrodes applied to one or both temples

B. Useful most frequently with affective disorders, especially depression unresponsive to medications and some behaviors of schizophrenic disorder

C. Six to ten treatments administered over 2 to 4 weeks

D. Two to three times per week

E. Nursing considerations
   1. Avoid use of term "shock" therapy
   2. Many clients experience fear
   3. Client must sign consent form

E. Indications
  1. Emergency therapy for suicidal client
  2. Affective disorder unresponsive to medications
  3. Clients who are unable to take medications because of pregnancy or cardiac status
  4. Catatonic stupor or excitement

G. Administration of ECT
  1. 100% oxygen given—preparation for apnea during seizure
  2. Muscle relaxants given—Anectine
  3. Anesthesia given—short-acting barbiturate
  4. Atropine sulfate given to dry secretions so client does not choke
  5. Bite block applied into mouth to prevent breaking of teeth and biting of tongue
  6. Electrodes placed bilateral or unilateral on temples
  7. Done in operating room or in a specially equipped room

H. Complications
  1. Increased intracerebral pressure
  2. Spontaneous fractures—usually decreased incidence now because of muscle relaxants being used
  3. Cardiac complications—usually related to anesthesia

I. Side effects
  1. Temporary confusion
  2. Temporary amnesia
  3. Headaches—treat with medications
  4. Agitation
  5. Postural hypotension
  6. Nausea
  7. Muscle soreness
  8. Fatigue
  9. Somnolence

J. Nursing interventions post-ECT
  1. Maintain patent airway
  2. Suction if required
  3. Position on side
     a. Prevents aspiration
     b. Prevents or deals with vomiting
  4. Closely monitor vital signs
  5. Provide orientation
  6. Assist with ambulation
  7. Administer antianxiety agents for agitation
  8. Administer antiemetics for nausea

IV. Orthomolecular therapy

A. Definition: nutritional therapy
B. Use of food and nutrients
   1. Maintain health
   2. Treat disease
   3. Support medical care
C. Megavitamin therapy
   1. Used for schizophrenia
   2. Theory
      a. Have requirements for nutrients that food alone cannot meet
      b. Value is controversial
      c. Unsubstantiated by scientific evidence

V. Psychopharmacology

A. Role of the nurse
   1. Conduct a baseline assessment of the client
   2. Provide client education
   3. Monitor drug effects
      a. Behavioral changes
      b. Therapeutic value
      c. Side effects
      d. Adverse reactions
   4. Administer medications
   5. Coordinate treatment modalities
B. Medication assessment guideline: obtain information about any past medications taken by the client
   1. Name of drug
   2. Reason prescribed
   3. Length of time taken
   4. Highest daily dose
   5. Was it effective?
   6. Side effects or adverse reactions
   7. Was it taken as prescribed? If not—why?
C. Drug interactions: risk factors for increased drug interactions
   1. Polypharmacy
   2. High doses
   3. Geriatric clients
   4. Inadequate client education
   5. Concurrent illness
   6. Risk for overdose

D. **Antianxiety agents**
    1. Common indications
       a. Anxiety
       b. Sleep
       c. Muscle spasms
       d. Seizure disorders
       e. Neuroleptic—induced akathisia (client cannot stay still, pacing, restlessness)
       f. Alcohol withdrawal
    2. Types, side effects, nursing implications (Table 6-2)
E. **Antidepressant drugs**
    1. Common indications for use (Table 6-3)
       a. Major depressive illness: unipolar and bipolar
       b. Panic disorder
       c. Enuresis in children
       d. Bulimia (Prozac)
       e. Obsessive-compulsive disorder (Anafranil)
    2. Types, dosage, actions, side effects, and nursing implications (Table 6-4)
       a. Tricyclic antidepressants
          (1) Intoxication syndrome or overdose symptoms
             (a) Hallucinations
             (b) Delirium
             (c) Agitation
             (d) Sensitivity to sounds
             (e) Dilated pupils
             (f) Hypothermia
             (g) Hyperpyrexia
             (h) Seizures
             (i) Coma
             (j) Dysrhythmias, especially tachycardias
             (k) Respiratory arrest
          (2) Treatment for intoxication or overdose
             (a) Induce emesis
             (b) Perform gastric lavage
             (c) Provide cardiac monitoring
             (d) Initiate respiratory support
             (e) Obtain arterial blood gases
             (f) Administer
                (i) Physostigmine
                (ii) Valium

Table 6-2. Antianxiety Agents

Types	Oral Dosages mg/day	Actions	Side Effects	Nursing Implications	Withdrawal Syndromes
Benzodiazepines					
Xanax (Alprazolam)	0.5-4	Wide range in central nervous system	Drowsiness	Advise client to use caution when using equipment or driving car	*Mild:* Tremulousness
Librium (Chlordiazepoxide)	20-100	Antianxiety Anticonvulsant	Sedation Ataxia Dizziness		Insomnia Dizziness Headaches
Tranxene (Chlorazepate)	7.5-60	Skeletal muscle relaxant	Feelings of detachment	Prevent falls, use caution with activity	Tinnitus Anorexia
Valium (Diazepam)	10-40	Hypnotic effects Potentiates inhibitory	Increased irritability or	Discourage social isolation	Vertigo Blurred vision
Ativan (Lorazepam)	2-6	neurotransmitter GABA	hostility Rebound	Observe for lack of control over	Agitation Anxiety
Serax (Oxazepam)	15-90	Blocks cortical and limbic arousal	insomnia Paradoxical	impulses In short-term use,	*Severe:* Diarrhea
Klonopin (Clonazepam)	1.5-2		excitement in the older adult or the debilitated	slowly taper off Implement weight control measures	Hypotension Hyperthermia Neuromuscular
			Increased appetite Weight gain	Advise client to take with meals Dose decreased if	Irritability Psychosis Seizures
			Nausea Headache Confusion	nausea, confusion, depression Give mild analgesia	
			Depression Pruritus Skin rashes	if headache Monitor and report pruritis Rashes not usually significant	

Nonbenzodiazepines					
Buspar	10-40	Less sedation than with benzodiazepines No skeletal muscle relaxation No anticonvulsant activity Not effective in alcohol abuse	No interaction with CNS depressants	Same as with benzodiazepines	No physical dependence
Antihistamines					
Benedryl Atarax	50 300	Antianxiety Antihistamine Antiemetic sedative	Lowers seizure threshold	Observe for seizure activity Advise client to stop driving	No physical dependence
Nonbarbiturate Sedatives/ Hypnotics					
Dalmane (Flurazepam) Halcion (Triazolam) Restoril (Temazepam)	15-30 0.25-.5 15-30	Various degrees of central nervous system depression Sedatives decrease anxiety and produce relaxation Hypnotics produce sleep Do not significantly reduce REM sleep Facilitate the action of inhibitory neurotransmitter GAGA (ganna-aminobutyric acid) Loci of action—limbic, thalamus, midbrain reticular formation		See Benzodiazepines	

Table 6-3. Predictors of Antidepressant Response

Tricyclics	MAOI
Positive predictors	**Positive predictors**
Anorexia	Hypochondriasis
Weight loss	Somatic anxiety
Insomnia (middle and late)	Irritability
Diurnal mood swing	Agoraphobia
Psychomotor retardation	Social phobias
Agitation	Anergia
Decreased functioning	Hysterical traits
Acute onset	Bipolar disorder
Family history of depression	Unresponsive to other
Self and family history of	antidepressants
drug responsiveness	
Therapeutic blood levels of	
antidepressants	
Agoraphobia	
Negative predictors	**Negative predictors**
Presence of other psychiatric	Depressed mood
disturbances	Guilt
Chronic symptoms	Ideas of reference
Psychotic features	Nihilistic delusions
Predominant somatic symptoms	Affective personality disorders
Previous unsuccessful drug	
trials	
Previous sensitivity or	
adverse reactions	

Modified from Schoonover SC: In *Bassuk EL,* Schoonover SC and Gelenberg AJ, editors: *The practitioner's guide to psychoactive drugs,* ed 2, New York & London, 1984, Plenum Medical Books Co. and Nardil: Parke-Davis Product Monograph, ed 4, Morris Plains, N.J., 1982, Parke-Davis, Medical Affairs Department.(From Stuart and Sundeen, 1991, p. 712.)
From Stuart G, Sundeen S: *Principles and practice of psychiatric nursing,* ed 4, St Louis, 1991, Mosby.

      (iii) Mannitol
      (iv) Lidocaine
  b. Monoamine oxidase inhibitors
    (1) Action—block the action of monoamine oxidase, an enzyme that deactivates norepinephrine, dopamine, and serotonin in the central nervous system
    (2) Common drugs
       (a) Isocarboxazid (Marplan)—30 to 70 mg/day
       (b) Phenelzine (Nardil)—45 to 90 mg/day
       (c) Trenyclypromine (Parnate)—20 to 60 mg/day

Table 6-4. Antidepressant Medications

Types	Oral Dosages mg/day	Actions	Side Effects	Nursing Implications	Withdrawal Syndromes	Contrain-dications
Tricyclic						
Amitriptyline (Elavil)	50-300	Block reuptake of neuro-transmitters (serotonin, norepineph-rine) at the presynaptic neuron Take 3 to 4 weeks to reach the therapeutic level	*Anticholinergic:* Dry mouth Constipation Tachycardia Blurred vision Urinary retention *Sympathetic nervous system:* Insomnia Confusion Dizziness Postural hypotension Nervousness Tremors	Encourage: Hydration Sugar-free mouth lozenges High-fiber foods Stool softeners Tolerance can develop after a few weeks Take vital signs while sitting and standing one-half hour after dose, have client rise slowly and dangle feet before standing	Malaise Muscle aches Chills Nausea Dizziness Anxiety	Avoid during acute recovery after a myocardial infarction Clients with history of cardiovascular disorders require careful monitoring Careful consideration with seizure disorders
Doxepin (Adapin, Sinequan)	50-300					
Imipramine (Tofranil)	50-300					
Chlomipramine (Anafranil)	50-250					
Desipramine (Norpramin, Pertofrane)	50-300					
Nortriptyline (Aventyl, Pamelar)	50-150					
Protriptyline	15-60					

Continued.

Table 6-4. Antidepressant Medications

Types	Oral Dosages mg/day	Actions	Side Effects	Nursing Implications	Withdrawal Syndromes	Contrain-dications
Tricyclic —cont'd			*Central nervous system:* Drowsiness Sedation Extrapyramidal symptoms (see antipsychotics) *Cardiovascular:* Tachycardia ECG changes: QRS and QT interval prolongation Sudden death Clients at risk for cardiac heart block: over 50, family history of heart disease, preexisting cardiac disease, bundle-branch block	Advise client to use caution in operating machinery or driving Administer at bedtime Take a careful cardiac history Do a pretreatment ECG, especially in clients over 40 years of age		Lowers seizure threshold Bipolar disorder with rapid cycling between mania and depression

	Dosage	Action/Use	Side Effects	Nursing Considerations	Comments
Selective Serotonin Reuptake Inhibitors Paxil (Paroxetine HC1)	20-50	Inhibition of neuronal reuptake of serotonin Treatment of major depression	No significant ECG changes Headache Abdominal Pain Fever Chest pain Back pain Palpitations Diaphoresis Ejaculatory disturbance Nausea Dry mouth Constipation Dizziness Insomnia Nervousness Pharyngitis Upper respiratory infection	Caution client about operating hazardous machinery and driving Advise to check with doctor if taking any over-the-counter medications Advise client to avoid alcohol Inform client to notify physician if pregnant or breast-feeding Administer in single daily dose, usually in morning	No demon-strated physical dependence	Not recommended in combination with Tryptophan (headache, nausea, sweat-ing, dizziness) Do not combine with MAO inhibitors, as fatal reactions have occurred (hyperthermia, rigidity, myoclonus, autonomic instability, delirium, coma)
Others Prozac Zoloft (see p. 109)						

(3) Indication—treat depression that has not responded to tricyclics
(4) Side effects/adverse reactions
    (a) CNS effects
        (i) Anxiety
        (ii) Agitation
        (iii) Dizziness
        (iv) Drowsiness
        (v) Euphoria
        (vi) Headache
        (vii) Muscle twitching
        (viii) Weakness
    (b) Anticholinergic effects
        (i) Dry mouth
        (ii) Blurred vision
        (iii) Constipation
    (c) Hypotension
    (d) Anginal pain
    (e) Leukopenia
(5) Interactions
    (a) Hypertensive crises when taken with foods containing tyramine
        Foods to avoid
        (i) Cheese, especially aged or matured
        (ii) Protein, fermented or aged
        (iii) Beer, red wine, sherry, liquors, cognac
        (iv) Yeast or protein extracts
        (v) Fava or broad bean pods
        (vi) Beef or chicken liver
        (vii) Spoiled or overripe fruit
        (viii) Banana peel
        (ix) Yogurt
        Foods in moderation
        (i) Chocolate
        (ii) Sour cream
        (iii) Clear spirits and white wine
        (iv) Avocado
        (v) New Zealand spinach
        (vi) Soy sauce
        (vii) Caffeine drinks
        Medications to avoid
        (i) Decongestants

        (ii)   Allergy and hay fever remedies
       (iii) Narcotics
      (iv) Inhalants for asthma
       (v) Local anesthetics with epinephrine
      (vi) Weight-reducing pills
  (b) May cause hypoglycemia when used with hypoglycemic agents, both oral and SQ

c. Prozac (Fluoxetine)
  (1) Action—inhibition of CNS neuronal uptake of serotonin only
  (2) Indications
    (a) Depression
    (b) Obsessive-compulsive disorder
    (c) Bulimia
    (d) Obesity
  (3) Dosage—20 to 80 mg/day
  (4) Side effects/adverse reactions
    (a) Anxiety
    (b) Insomnia
    (c) Anorexia
    (d) Tremors
    (e) Rash—may develop into systemic reaction
    (f) Increased suicidal ideation
  (5) Binds to protein—may interfere with plasma levels of other protein-binding drugs
    (a) Digoxin
    (b) Coumadin

d. Zoloft
  (1) Action—serotonin reuptake inhibitor
  (2) Indication: agitated depression
  (3) Dosage—50 to 200 mg/day
  (4) Side effects/adverse reactions
    (a) Nausea
    (b) Diarrhea
    (c) Dry mouth
    (d) Insomnia
    (e) Ejaculatory delay
    (f) Few cardiac effects—no significant ECG, heart rate, or conduction changes
    (g) Wide margins of safety in overdosage

   e. Mood stabilizing drugs
      (1) Lithium—natural occurring salt
         (a) Used in treatment of cyclical affective disorders,
            especially bipolar illness
         (b) Action—theories
            (i) Corrects ion exchange
            (ii) Alters sodium transport
            (iii) Normalizes synaptic neurotransmission
               of norepinephrine, serotonin, and
               dopamine
            (iv) Changes receptor sensitivity for serotonin
         (c) Pretreatment assessment
            (i) Thyroid studies
            (ii) Renal—urinalysis, 24-hour creatinine
               clearance, creatinine, BUN, electrolytes
         (d) Types of lithium (Table 6-5)
         (e) Lithium therapy dosage
            (i) 300 mg TID until steady state—
               approximately 7 days
            (ii) Takes up to 4 weeks to have a therapeutic
               effect
            (iii) Levels
               ▼ Therapeutic—0.6 to 1.5 mEq/liter
               ▼ Toxicity—greater than
                  2.0 mEq/liter
               ▼ Lethal—greater than 2.5 mEq/liter

Table 6-5. Types of Lithium

Generic Name	Trade Name	Available Tablets
Lithium carbonate	Eskalith PF1–Lith Lithotabs Lithene Lithonate	150, 300 mg
Lithium carbonate, sustained-release	Lithobid Eskalith C-R	300 mg 450 mg
Lithium citrate, concentrate	Ciba-Lith Lithonate-S	5 mg/300 mg

Laraia M, and Stuart G: *Quick psychopharmacology reference,* St Louis, 1991, Mosby.

        (iv) Reassess blood level every 5 days initially for 1 month, then every 3 to 6 months

(f) Side effects
- (i) Fine hand tremors (50% of clients)
- (ii) Weight gain (60% of clients)
- (iii) Polyuria (60% of clients)
- (iv) Gastric irritation
- (v) Anorexia
- (vi) Abdominal cramps
- (vii) Mild nausea
- (viii) Lethargy

(g) Long-term adverse effects
- (i) Hypothyroidism
- (ii) Mild diabetes mellitus
- (iii) Nephrogenic diabetes insipidus

(h) Lithium toxicity clinical findings
- (i) Greater than 2.0 mEq/liter
  - ▼ Anorexia
  - ▼ Nausea
  - ▼ Vomiting
  - ▼ Dysarthria
  - ▼ Course hand tremors
  - ▼ Twitching
  - ▼ Weakness
  - ▼ Ataxia
  - ▼ Tinnitus
  - ▼ Vertigo
  - ▼ Drowsiness
  - ▼ Lethargy

(i) Lithium intoxication—lethal level
- (i) Greater than 2.5 mEq/Liter
  - ▼ Fever
  - ▼ Decreased urine output
  - ▼ Decreased BP
  - ▼ ECG changes
  - ▼ Seizures
  - ▼ Coma
  - ▼ Death

(j) Causes for increase in lithium level
- (i) Decreased sodium intake
- (ii) Diuretic therapy
- (iii) Decreased renal functioning

         (iv) Sweating

         (v) Diarrhea

         (vi) Dehydration

         (vii) Vomiting

         (viii) Overdose

    (k) Ways to maintain lithium level

         (i) Dividing doses

         (ii) Adequate sodium intake

         (iii) Adequate fluid intake—2 to 3 liters/day

         (iv) Monitor side effects and toxic effects

    (l) Management of toxicity

         (i) Hold lithium

         (ii) Obtain lithium blood level

         (iii) Electrocardiogram

         (iv) Vital signs

         (v) Hydrate—5 to 6 liters/day

         (vi) If overdose—emetic, nasogastric suction

         (vii) Increase clearance with

             ▼ Aminophylline IV

             ▼ IV sodium lactate

             ▼ Intake of NaCl

             ▼ Osmotic diuresis—urea or mannitol, IV

             ▼ Peritoneal dialysis or hemodialysis

  (2) Tegretol

    (a) Primary clinical indication is for prevention of temporal lobe epilepsy, but it has been found to be a mood stabilizer in affective disorders

    (b) Takes effect in 10 days

    (c) Side effects

         (i) Skin rash

         (ii) Sore throat

         (iii) Low-grade fever

         (iv) Drowsiness

         (v) Vertigo

         (vi) Ataxia

         (vii) Diplopia

         (viii) 25% decrease in WBC

         (ix) Agranulocytosis—rare but irreversible

F. Antipsychotic drugs

  1. Actions

      a. Dopamine antagonists

      b. Block dopamine receptors

2. Indications

      a. Schizophrenia

      b. Organic brain syndrome with psychosis

      c. Severe depression with psychotic features

      d. Manic phase of bipolar disorder

      e. Vomiting

      f. Vertigo

      g. Enhancement of analgesics for pain relief

      h. Huntington's disease

      i. La Tourrette disorder

3. Target symptoms that require treatment

      a. Hyperactivity

      b. Poor motivation

      c. Flat affect

      d. Anxiety

      e. Agitation

      f. Withdrawal

      g. Loose associations

      h. Delusions

      i. Hallucinations

      j. Paranoia

      k. Negativism

4. Common antipsychotic drugs and dosages

      a. Chlorpromazine (Thorazine)—300 to 1400 mg/day

      b. Thioridazine (Mellaril)—300 to 800 mg/day

      c. Mesordazine (Serentil)—100 to 500 mg/day

      d. Perphenezine (Trilafon)—8 to 64 mg/day

      e. Trifluoperazine (Stelazine)—10 to 80 mg/day

      f. Fluphenazine (Prolixin)—5 to 40 mg/day

      g. Thiothixene (Navane)—10 to 60 mg/day

      h. Haloperidol (Haldol)—5 to 100 mg/day

      i. Loxapine (Loxitane)—50 to 250 mg/day

      j. Molindane (Moban)—25 to 250 mg/day

      k. Clozapine (Clozaril)—300 to 600 mg/day

      l. Risperidone (Risperdal)—4 to 6 mg/day

       (Laraia and Stuart, 1991)

5. Side effects/adverse reactions/treatment and nursing implications (Table 6-6 and Box 6-2)

Table 6-6. Side Effects and Adverse Reactions of Antipsychotic Drugs

Side Effects/Adverse Reactions	Treatment and Nursing Implications
Neurological	
Extrapyramidal Symptoms (EPS) ▼ Acute dystonic reactions: occur suddenly and are frightening; spasms of major muscle groups of neck, back, eyes; respiratory compromise	Administer anticholinergic, dopaminergic, or gagaminergic drugs (see Box 16-2, p. 117) Have respiratory support equipment available
▼ Akathisia: client cannot remain still; pacing, restlessness	Rule out anxiety or agitation

▼ Parkinson's syndrome
   a. Akinesia—absence or slowness of motion
   b. Cogwheel rigidity of elbow and muscle stiffness
   c. Fine tremor—"pill rolling" motion of fingers
	Add an antidyskinetic drug such as Cogentin or Artane for 3 months and then taper (see Box 16-2, p. 117)

▼ Seizures: usually grand mal, no warning aura, lower seizure threshold	Decrease dose; anticonvulsants do not protect nonseizure disorder clients
▼ Tardive dyskinesia (TD): tongue protrusion, lip smacking, puckering, sucking, chewing, blinking, lateral jaw movements, grimacing, choreiform movements of the limbs and trunk, shoulders shrugging, pelvic thrusting, wrist and ankle flexion or rotation, foot tapping, toe movements, stereotyped involuntary movements, which may be mild or severely crippling	May need soft foods and soft shoes for feet movements Good denture care Velcro closures on clothing and shoes There is no treatment for TD, though several drugs are in the experimental stages May be irreversible, especially if not discovered early and if antipsychotic drugs cannot be stopped Monitor for symptoms
Autonomic Nervous System	
Anticholinergic side effects ▼ Blurred vision ▼ Constipation ▼ Tachycardia ▼ Urinary retention ▼ Decreased sweating and salivation	Tolerance develops in days to weeks *Treat symptomatically:* Sugarless candy and gum; Bulk diets; Stool softeners; Fluids; Exercise; Cholinergic agonist, Bethanechol (Urecholine), for urinary retention

Table 6-6. Side Effects and Adverse Reactions of Antipsychotic Drugs—cont'd

Side Effects/Adverse Reactions	Treatment and Nursing Implications
Cardiovascular	
▼ Orthostatic hypotension with dizziness, tachycardia: drop in diastolic BP by greater than 20 mm/Hg with a change in position from lying to sitting or sitting to standing ▼ ECG abnormalities	Monitor BP Increased fluid intake to expand vascular volume Have client rise slowly and dangle feet while sitting Have client wear support hose Baseline and follow up ECG and vital sign monitoring for patients with preexisting cardiac disease
Dermatologic	
▼ Systemic dermatosis Maculopapular erythematous Itchy rash on face Neck Chest, extremities ▼ Photosensitivity Sever sunburn	Discontinue drug and start again cautiously when rash disappears Change to a drug in another chemical class Topical steroids if necessary Lower dose Use sunscreen and wear clothing on overexposed areas
Hematologic	
Agranulocytosis develops abruptly; accompanied by fever, malaise, ulcerative sore throat, leukopenia (WBC under 5000)	*Extreme emergency:* Be alert for high fever and ulcerative sore throat, particularly in geriatric females Monitor WBC If occurs, discontinue drug immediately and initiate reverse isolation Antibiotics when appropriate
Hepatic	
▼ Jaundice ▼ Fever ▼ Nausea ▼ Abdominal pain ▼ Malaise ▼ Pruritus ▼ Abnormal liver function tests— ALT, AST	Discontinue drug Is reversible and self-limiting Bed rest High-protein/carbohydrate, low-fat diet

Continued.

Table 6-6. Side Effects and Adverse Reactions of Antipsychotic Drugs—cont'd

Side Effects/Adverse Reactions	Treatment and Nursing Implications
Endocrine	
▼ Galactorrhea	Decrease dose or change drug
▼ Amenorrhea	Partial tolerance may develop
▼ Breast enlargement and engorgement	Be sure that female clients are not actually pregnant
▼ Decreased libido	Diet and exercise regimen for weight gain
▼ Ejaculatory incompetence	
▼ Appetite increase and weight gain	Periodic breast exams, especially if personal or family history of breast cancer
▼ Hypothermia or hyperthermia	
▼ False positive pregnancy test	
Ophthalmologic	
Toxic pigmentary retinopathy—client notices brownish discoloration of vision, loss of visual acuity, possible blindness	Degenerative and irreversible Avoidable Particularly related to doses of thioridazine (Mellaril) over 800 mg/day Never give above 800 mg/day
Neuroleptic Malignant Syndrome	
▼ High fever	*Extreme emergency:*
▼ Tachycardia	Early recognition is critical
▼ Muscle rigidity	Avoid marked dehydration in all patients
▼ Stupor	
▼ Tremor	Discontinue all drugs immediately
▼ Incontinence	Provide nutrition and hydration
▼ Leukocytosis	Renal dialysis for renal failure
▼ Elevated serum CPK	Ventilation for acute respiratory failure
▼ Hyperkalemia	
▼ Renal failure	Reduction of fever
▼ Increased pulse and respirations	
▼ Sweating	

Modified from Stuart G and Sundeen S: *Principles and practice of psychiatric nursing,* ed 5, St Louis, 1995, Mosby.

Box 6-2. Drugs to Treat Extrapyramidal Side Effects

Anticholinergic
  Benztropine mesylate (Cogentin)
  Trihexyphenidyl (Artane)
  Biperiden (Akineton)
  Procyclidine (Kemadrin)
  Diphenhydramine (Benadryl)
Dopaminergic
  Amantadine (Symmetrel)
Gabaminergic
  Diazepam (Valium)
  Lorazepam (Ativan)

6. Clozapine (Clozaril)
   a. Acts selectively on D_1 receptors
   b. Low potency, sedating agent
   c. Works on both positive and negative symptoms of schizophrenia
   d. Few extrapyramidal symptoms
   e. Dosage 250 to 450 mg per day
   f. Believed not to cause tardive dyskinesia
   g. Side effects/adverse reactions/incidence
      (1) Sedation and fatigue (34% to 58%)
      (2) Weight gain (34% to 63%)
      (3) Gastrointestinal symptoms (17% to 40%)
      (4) Hypotension (11% to 23%)
      (5) Tachycardia (7% to 14%)
      (6) Fever (5% to 9%)
      (7) Seizures (4%)
      (8) ECG changes (2% to 4%)
      (9) Leukopenia or agranulocytosis (1% to 3%)
   h. Frequent lab work for liver function (ALT, AST) and for agranulocytosis is indicated, which increases significantly the expense of the drug therapy
7. Risperidone (Risperdal)
   a. Action—dopamine type 2 and serotonin type 2 antagonism
   b. Has decreased incidence of agranulocytosis
   c. Frequent lab work not necessary, which decreases cost of therapy
   d. Side effects
      (1) Neuroleptic malignant syndrome

   (2) Tardive dyskinesia (most often in the older adult)

   (3) Lengthens QT interval on the ECG

   (4) Orthostatic hypotension

   (5) Cognitive and motor impairment

   (6) Weight gain

  e. Dosage—4 to 6 mg/day on BID basis

  f. Side effects/adverse reactions similar to the antipsychotics

   (1) Sleepiness

   (2) Increased duration of sleep

   (3) Orthostatic hypotension

   (4) Weight gain

   (5) Erectile and ejaculatory dysfunction

   (6) Tachycardia

   (7) Low incidence of extrapyramidal symptoms (16%)

   (8) No documentation of agranulocytosis

REVIEW QUESTIONS

1. In crisis intervention what technique might be used that is inappropriate in traditional therapy?
   a. Counseling
   b. Humor
   c. Advice-giving
   d. Theme identification

2. The psychiatric nurse is talking to a group of business owners about maturational events and crises. How would the nurse answer the question about when involutional depression is most common?
   a. In women before age of 47
   b. In men aged 50 to 58
   c. In persons poorly adjusted to middle age
   d. Following endocrine changes of middle age

3. An actively psychotic client is being assessed by the nurse for participation in a milieu group. Which is the most appropriate group for this client?
   a. A highly structured, task-oriented group
   b. An activity group
   c. A group is not appropriate
   d. A movement therapy group, after a short period of isolation

4. The role of the nurse in environmental therapy includes
   a. Coordinating team activities, maintaining the environment 24 hours per day
   b. Referring others to work with families, observing in groups
   c. Coordinating medical care, selecting programs
   d. Observing community meetings, leading groups

5. A student nurse is discussing the purposes of psychodrama with the nurse. Which statement about psychodrama by the student indicates a need for further discussion?
   a. Clients can dramatize past and present relationships
   b. It provides opportunities for clients to gain insight into conflicts
   c. It helps schizophrenics get in touch with their feelings
   d. It promotes an opportunity for the catharsis of feelings

6. The activity therapy the nurse would select to promote reminiscing in a group aged over 70 is
   a. Poetry
   b. Art
   c. Movement
   d. Music

7. Professional preparation for a nurse wanting to lead a therapeutic group would include
   a. A Bachelor's degree in nursing with course work in group process
   b. A strong commitment to understand the group process
   c. Attendance at yearly in-services for group process updates
   d. A Master's degree with supervision as a group leader

8. In the initial stage of group development, the least common characteristic is that
   a. Group members look to the leader for structure, approval, and acceptance
   b. Group members decide if the group will be of a closed or open status
   c. Subgroups form within the group
   d. Group members accept their individual differences

9. A client seeks counseling from the nurse for marital conflict that includes a history of physical abuse. What would be the initial intervention in this client's plan of care?
   a. Assist the client in identifying aspects of the client's life that are under the control of the client
   b. Facilitate the client's desire to gain knowledge of the democratic family process
   c. Discuss issues of the use of stereotypic gender role behavior and the effect of violence in the family
   d. Explain theories of family violence so the client understands patterns in the marital conflict

10. Which documentation finding would indicate that a family had functional characteristics?
    a. Members are self-centered, and they use clear communication
    b. Boundaries are with minimal outside contacts
    c. Roles are fused
    d. Generational boundaries are present, with differences among members encouraged

11. A client is to receive his first electro-convulsive treatment (ECT). He states, "I'm afraid because my roommate told me I'll forget everything and my memory will never return." What is the best response?
    a. "Don't worry about it; you will get your memory back"
    b. "You may not experience memory loss, but you still need ECT to get better"
    c. "It may be best if you can't remember certain things"
    d. "There is memory loss, but it will return over a 2- to 3-week period"

12. Based on knowledge of electro-convulsive treatment, the nurse explains to the student nurse that atropine is given before the procedure primarily to
    a. Minimize intestinal contractions
    b. Decrease anxiety
    c. Dry up body secretions
    d. Prevent aspiration

13. Lithium, the drug of choice for bipolar disorders, has a narrow therapeutic range of
    a. 0.5 mEq/L to 1.5 mEq/L
    b. 0.6 mEq/L to 1.0 mEq/L
    c. 0.7 mEq/L to 1.3 mEq/L
    d. 1.0 mEq/L to 2.0 mEq/L

14. A client is receiving monoamine oxidase inhibitors (MAOs) as part of the treatment. Which food would be most important for the nurse to stress to avoid?
    a. Organ meats
    b. Sardines
    c. Shellfish
    d. Legumes

15. A client receiving lithium carbonate complains of blurred vision and appears confused. The nurse also notices that the client is having difficulty maintaining balance. Which of these nursing actions are appropriate?
    a. Administer a PRN antiparkinsonism drug and hold all other drugs
    b. Take the client's vital signs and administer high-potassium foods
    c. Hold the client's next dose of medication and notify the physician immediately
    d. Sit with client to talk and teach the side effects of lithium

16. Many of the major tranquilizers display untoward side effects. The one side effect displaying irreversible abnormal, involuntary movements of the tongue and mouth is
    a. Akathisia
    b. Tardive dyskinesia
    c. Agranulocytosis
    d. Dystonia

ANSWERS, RATIONALES, AND TEST-TAKING TIPS

Rationales	Test-Taking Tips

1. **Correct answer: c**

During a crisis the nurse must be creative and flexible while considering possible solutions for the client to consider. Giving advice is an active role, and it is permissible so that time spent in therapy may be decreased.

The approach is to read carefully to note that the question is asking about a technique that is "inappropriate" in traditional therapy. In this type of question make a selection, then carefully reread the question and your selection.

2. **Correct answer: c**

Involutional depression is a depression from within the person and not the result of external events. Note that this is a general question, so the correct option is more global than the others. Another way to look at this is that options *a, b,* and *c* could be listed as subcomponents of *d.*

If you have no idea of the correct answer, cluster options *a, b,* and *d* for being specific. Option *c* presents a general answer when it speaks of "persons."

3. **Correct answer: c**

If the client is actively psychotic, the groups given in the options are not appropriate.

The key words in the stem are "actively psychotic."

4. **Correct answer: a**

Nurses have 24-hour responsibility for maintaining the environment in milieu therapy. Authority and accountability is shared by team members. In option *b* nurses work with families

To select the correct answer, *go with what you know*—that nurses maintain the environment day to day—select option *a.* If you aren't sure of the other options, don't select them.

and also lead the groups. In option *c* nurses do coordinate medical care; they plan programs rather than select programs. In option *d* nurses participate in community meetings.

5. **Correct answer: c**

Schizophrenics may have increased psychotic symptoms, confuse "process" with reality, and become overwhelmed by unconscious material when psychodrama is incorporated into their activity therapy. Psychodrama should be used cautiously with these clients. The other options are purposes of psychodrama.

First note the key words, "indicates a need for further discussion." Look for an incorrect statement. If you still have no idea of the correct answer, note that option *c* is the only response with a specific type of client. The other options have a general focus. Select *c*.

6. **Correct answer: d**

Music therapy allows for reminiscing when old songs are played, since the long-term memory of the older adults is more functional than the short-term memory. The other therapies in options *a*, *b*, and *c* are not typically used for reminisce therapy.

Use a common sense approach to select *d*, since music would be the most likely activity for which a large group of people would have the most common background, especially for the melody or lyrics.

7. **Correct answer: d**

Nurses with a Master's degree in nursing, with an emphasis on group therapy training during their education and supervised training after their education are the most qualified to lead therapeutic groups.

The key words in the other options make them incorrect: in option *a* "course work" does not indicate a functional ability to lead groups; in option *b* "an understanding" does not validate application ability to group process; in option *c* "attendance at yearly updates" does not confirm that one has demonstrated abilities in group process. Option *d* is the only response that indicates an application of the knowledge of the nurse with groups.

8. Correct answer: b

Usually the leader decides if the group is to have an open or closed status in the pregroup stage of group formation. The other options are part of the initial stage, which is actually the second stage of group development.

If you have no idea of the correct answer, note that options *a, c,* and *d* indicate some type of interaction or process between the group members and/or the leader. Option *b* illustrates group action about an issue, the status. Select option *b.*

9. Correct answer: a

In dysfunctional families, roles are commonly fused, individualism is discouraged, and conflict is seen as negative. Interventions for dysfunctional families are focused on setting limits on acting-out behavior, getting family members to use *I* statements, and encouraging the use of community resources. By helping the client identify some aspects of life that are under the client's control, the nurse is attempting to move the client toward appropriate separateness. The other options focus on educational interventions inappropriate at this time. Option *b* assumes a client desire, and no information in the stem supports this option.

If you have no idea of the correct answer, cluster options *b, c,* and *d* under the headings of educational interventions, or you can think of it as the client's assuming a passive role. Select option *a* in which the client has to be active in a counseling session.

10. Correct answer: d

Option *d* is the most positive description of the four options. The other options are characteristics of dysfunctional families except for the aspect of clear communication. Communication in dysfunctional families has characteristics of being cold and distant. In functional families, communication is clear.

Note that options *a, b,* and *c* have a negative connotation, which lends to more dysfunctional rather than functional family characteristics. Reread the question and select *d*.

11. Correct answer: d

Many clients experience confusion and short-term memory loss with ECT. The memory loss clears 2 to 3 weeks after the last treatment. Eliminate the options *a, b* and *d,* which have parts of these statements as barriers to communication: in option *a* the phrase "don't worry" is giving reassurance; option *b* ("you need . . . to get better") and option *c* ("it may be best") are giving advice.

The best response shows honesty and informs the client based on facts, not feelings or thoughts of the nurse. To prepare for your exam, you may want to review either the barriers to communication or the therapeutic responses, rather than both, which might result in confusion.

12. Correct answer: c

Atropine is given 1 hour before treatment to reduce oral and gastric secretions so the client does not choke or aspirate. Option *d* may be considered a secondary

The approach is, *go with what you know.* Recall that atropine is an anticholinergic given before surgery to dry up secretions.

action of the effects of the atropine. Anesthesia, a short-acting barbiturate, is usually given to decrease anxiety and memory of the event. Atropine decreases intestinal and urinary peristalsis rather than minimize contractions.

13. **Correct answer: b**

A lithium level < 0.5 mEq/L will not be effective in relieving symptoms. A level greater than 2 mEq/L is considered in the toxic range, and a level > 2 mEq/L is considered life threatening.

Associate the therapeutic digoxin level with lithium: both are .5 to 2.0 as a maximum before becoming lethal or life threatening.

14. **Correct answer: b**

Food rich in tyramine (e.g., sardines), if not avoided, may cause a hypertensive crisis. The other foods listed are high in purines and are restricted in clients with gouty arthritis to minimize uric acid production.

The approach to this type of difficult question is to make your best educated guess. Remain calm. Take a few deep breaths and go on to the next question. Avoid an emotional reaction.

15. **Correct answer: c**

The client is displaying the first signs of lithium toxicity. The medication should be held and a physician should be notified to obtain an order for a stat serum lithium level. The other actions are inappropriate.

First note that the findings are not the usual type of side effects. Use your knowledge and common sense to select "hold the dose and notify the physician."

16. **Correct answer: b**

Recall that the *t*ongue has *t*ardive movements as a side effect of tranquilizers. Akathisia is an inability to sit still or a continued restlessness. Agranulocytosis is a diminished number of granulocytes. Dystonia is an impairment of muscle tone, usually of the head, neck, or tongue.

Identify the key word in the stem, "movements." Of the given options, identify the only answer with a movement focus, option *b*. The "kine" is the clue that the word deals with movement.

Anxiety, Somatoform and Dissociative Disorders

STUDY OUTCOMES

After completing this chapter, the reader will be able to do the following:

- ▼ Define anxiety.
- ▼ Identify characteristics of the four levels of anxiety.
- ▼ Describe the nursing process as it relates to the various levels of anxiety.
- ▼ Describe theoretical foundations of anxiety.
- ▼ Discuss the psychopathology of anxiety, somatoform, and dissociative disorders.

KEY TERMS

Anxiety	Subjective, internal response to nonspecific stressors that threaten one's security or sense of self.
Compulsion	Uncontrollable impulse to perform an act.
Depersonalization	Perception and experience of self as changed or lost that creates a sense of nonreality.
Derealization	Perception of environment as being not real.
Hypochondriasis	Preoccupation with the fear of having a serious illness.
Malingering	Conscious use of nonexistent physical symptoms to escape responsibilities or expectations.
Obsession	Persistent, unwanted thought that is recognized as irrational.
Phobia	Irrational fear.

CONTENT REVIEW

I. Anxiety

A. What is it?
1. A normal response to stress
2. A warning of impending danger
3. A result of threats that may be misperceived or misinterpreted
4. A subjective, individual experience
5. Cannot be observed directly
6. Precedes new experiences
7. Is contagious interpersonally, including nurse-client, client-nurse
8. A threat to self-esteem or identity
9. Preservation of self is key
10. Results when someone's values are threatened

B. Theories of the origin of anxiety
1. Psychoanalytic view (Freud)—primary anxiety
   a. Trauma of birth
   b. Primary needs (food, oxygen) might not be satisfied
   c. Tension from external causes
2. Interpersonal view (Sullivan)
   a. Fear of disapproval is central
   b. Originates with the mother/infant bond
   c. Mild or moderate levels are expressed as anger
   d. Can become growth producing
   e. Amount of anxiety relates to level of self-esteem

3. Behavioral view
   a. Frustration caused by interference in reaching a goal, such as the loss of a job
   b. Desire to avoid pain
   c. Arises through conflict
C. Precipitants of anxiety
   1. Threats to physical integrity
      a. Lack of food, clothing
      b. Injury
      c. Illness
      d. Abuse
   2. Threats to self-system
      a. Identity
      b. Self-esteem
   3. Multicaused
      a. Interpersonal
      b. Behavioral
      c. Genetic
      d. Biological
D. Physiological behaviors indicative of anxiety
   1. Palpitations
   2. Tachycardia
   3. Increased blood pressure
   4. Faintness
   5. Rapid breathing
   6. Shortness of breath
   7. Lump in throat
   8. Choking sensation
   9. Startle reaction
   10. Insomnia
   11. Tremors
   12. Rigidity
   13. Pacing
   14. Weakness
   15. Loss of appetite
   16. Nausea
   17. Diarrhea
   18. Frequent urination
   19. Flushed face
   20. Increased perspiration
   21. Itching
   22. Hot and cold spells
   23. Pale face

E. **Psychological manifestations of anxiety—4 levels (Figure 7-1)**
   1. Mild
      a. Alert
      b. Perceptual field increased
      c. Can increase learning
      d. Can produce growth and creativity
   2. Moderate
      a. Perceptual field narrowed
      b. Focused on immediate concerns
      c. Selective in attention
   3. Severe
      a. Perceptual field greatly reduced
      b. Focused on a specific detail
      c. Behavior focused on relieving anxiety
      d. Needs direction to focus
      e. Feeling of something bad about to happen
   4. Panic
      a. Dread
      b. Terror
      c. Unable to do things, even with direction
      d. Increased motor activity

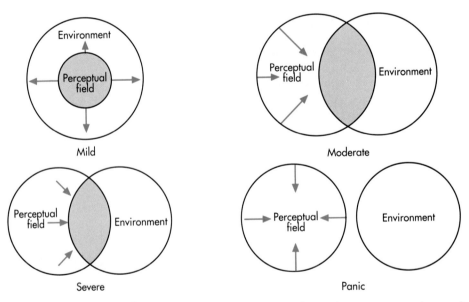

Figure 7-1. Levels of anxiety. (From Stuart G and Sundeen S: *Principles and practice of psychiatric nursing,* ed 5, St Louis, 1995, Mosby.)

    e. Distorted perceptions

    f. Loss of rational thought

    g. Inability to concentrate

    h. Decreased ability to relate to others

    i. Sense of impending doom

    j. If prolonged, leads to exhaustion and death

II. Anxiety disorders

    A. Generalized anxiety disorder—cause usually can be identified

       1. Unrealistic or excessive anxiety

       2. Physiological changes

       3. Dread of physical illness

       4. Fear that something unfortunate will happen

       5. Chronic muscular tension

       6. Restlessness

       7. Episodes of trembling and shakiness

       8. Chronic fatigue

       9. Dizziness

      10. Difficulty concentrating

      11. Irritability

      12. Sleep problems

      13. Do not recognize connection between anxiety and physical symptoms

      14. Focused on physical discomfort

    B. Panic disorders

       1. Intense episodes of anxiety appear intermittently—cause usually cannot be identified

       2. 5 to 30 minutes in length

       3. Symptoms of anxiety

       4. Sense of unreality

       5. Fear of dying

       6. Sense of going crazy

       7. Helplessness

       8. Feeling of being trapped

       9. Physical findings

          a. Choking sensation

          b. Labored breathing

          c. Pounding heart

          d. Chest pain

          e. Dizziness

          f. Nausea

        g. Blurred vision

        h. Numbness or tingling of extremities

   10. Develop anticipatory pattern of dread that attack will occur

        a. Hypervigilant

        b. Study body for sign of attack

        c. Increased constriction of lifestyle—avoidance of people and places

C. Phobic disorders

   1. Irrational fears of an object or situation

   2. Associated with panic-level anxiety

   3. Defense mechanisms

        a. Repression

        b. Displacement

   4. Agoraphobia

        a. Trapped in a situation with no escape

        b. Fear or sense of helplessness or embarrassment if attack occurs

        c. Fear of public places

            (1) Restaurants

            (2) Theaters

            (3) Malls

        d. Avoid situations

   5. Social phobia

        a. Fear of being critically evaluated by others

        b. Fear of making a fool of oneself

        c. Incidence—3% to 13%

D. Obsessive-compulsive disorder

   1. Obsessive thoughts involve violence, aggression, orderliness, sexual behavior, religion

   2. Thoughts are intrusive—uncontrollably interrupt conscious thought

   3. Interferes with ability to function

   4. Behavior patterns to decrease anxiety

   5. Behaviors are associated with obsessive thoughts

   6. Behaviors neutralize the thought

   7. During stressful times, ritualistic behavior increases

   8. Examples

        a. Washing hands

        b. Stirring coffee a certain number of times

        c. Hanging clothes in closet in certain direction and order

        d. Turning lights on and off

e. Addictive behaviors
(1) Shopping
(2) Gambling
(3) Binge eating
(4) Hypersexual behavior
9. Defense mechanisms
a. Repression
b. Displacement
c. Undoing
10. Example of process—compulsive bathing is "undoing" thoughts of sexual behavior
E. **Posttraumatic stress disorder**
1. Experience stress outside of normal life experience
a. Natural disaster
b. Combat
c. Rape
d. Automobile accident
e. Victim of crime/violence
f. Abuse—sexual, physical, emotional
2. Symptoms
a. Reexperiencing the event—flashbacks
b. Numbing of responsiveness
c. Reduced involvement with the external world
d. Depression
e. Anxiety
f. Nightmares
g. Dissociative episodes
h. Dissociative identity disorder
F. **Nursing process with anxiety disorders**
1. Assessment
a. Level of anxiety
b. Psychological and physical symptoms of anxiety
c. Safety issues
2. Nursing diagnoses related to anxiety
a. Ineffective individual coping
b. Sleep pattern disturbance
c. Self-esteem disturbance
d. Fear
e. Altered nutrition
f. Powerlessness
g. Impaired social interaction
h. Sensory-perceptual alterations

3. Client goals
   a. Are set mutually with client
   b. Must be measurable
   c. Must be realistic
   d. In severe or panic anxiety, goal is to reduce anxiety quickly
   e. Should relate to nursing diagnosis
   f. Client demonstrates a reduction or elimination of problematic behavior
   g. The client tolerates mild anxiety and uses it constructively
4. Interventions for general anxiety
   a. Establish trust
      (1) Listen
      (2) Answer questions
      (3) Provide unconditional acceptance
   b. Recognize anxiety
      (1) Link behaviors with anxiety
      (2) Link beginning of anxious feelings with precipitant of anxiety
   c. Protect the client
      (1) Monitor anxiety
      (2) Decrease stimulation
      (3) Do not force client into situations that provoke high anxiety
      (4) Do not attack coping mechanisms such as repetitive actions—stirring coffee, washing hands
   d. Modify the environment
      (1) Set limits
      (2) Limit interactions with others
      (3) Warm baths
      (4) Whirlpools
   e. Activity
      (1) An activity limits the amount of time for destructive behaviors
      (2) Vigorous activity decreases anxiety release
   f. Creative outlets
      (1) Art therapy
      (2) Music therapy
      (3) Journaling
   g. Medications—antianxiety
   h. Relaxation techniques (Table 7-1)

Table 7-1. **Relaxation Techniques**

Type	Process
▼ Meditation 　Visual—awareness of what is happening inside 　Auditory (Centering)—repetition of word or a group of words (MANTRA)	Concentrate on an object to exclusion of everything else Candle Flower Vase While repeating a word concentrate on 　▼ Breathing 　▼ Heartbeat
▼ Visualization—guided imagery	Picture self in favorite place, such as the seashore: see the waves, feel the breeze, feel the sun, taste the salt, experience all 5 senses for 3 to 5 minutes
▼ Desensitization	Meditation used with visualization to desensitize to a situation that causes stress. Break situation down into steps—with each step, utilize meditation and visualization
▼ Progressive relaxation	Systematically tense and relax various muscle groups for 15 to 45 seconds with each group and a total time of 20 to 30 minutes
▼ Autogenic training	Induces sensation of heaviness in limbs Sensation of warmth in limbs Concentrate on regular heartbeat Concentrate on regular respirations Sense of upper abdominal warmth Coolness in forehead

5. Interventions specific to the obsessive-compulsive disorder
   a. Do not interrupt compulsive behaviors
   b. Provide a schedule that distracts from behaviors
   c. Provide for safety related to behaviors, such as skin care for the hand washer
   d. Explore situations that precipitate the behavior
   e. Explore issues of low self-esteem

     6. Interventions specific to phobias
       a. Desensitization
       b. Insight into basis of anxiety
     7. Interventions specific to posttraumatic stress disorder
       a. Desensitization through gradual exposure to the event or situations similar to the event
       b. Individual therapy
         (1) Loss-of-control issues
         (2) Anger
       c. Group therapy—homogeneous (similar experiences)
       d. Hypnotherapy

III. Somatoform disorders

  A. **Somatoform disorders**
     1. Rule out physical illness first
     2. Clients focus anxiety on body symptoms
       a. Headaches
       b. Digestive upsets
       c. Aches and pains
     3. Client goals
       a. Develops appropriate concern about health status
       b. Decreases preoccupation with body functions and symptoms
       c. Develops interest in others and less interest in self
       d. Explores and revises sense of self
     4. Interventions by nurses
       a. Encourage client to recognize, label, and work through feelings and emotions
       b. Contract with client to engage in relationships with others to redirect interest
       c. Stimulate verbalization of anxiety and exploration of anxiety source
       d. Encourage the client the use of relaxation techniques as anxiety increases
  B. **Conversion disorder**
     1. Lost or altered body functioning related to psychological conflict or need
     2. Not intentionally produced
     3. No organic cause
     4. Example: bride wakes up the morning of wedding paralyzed from the waist down
     5. "La Belle Indifference"—unconcerned with symptoms. Example: she is not worried that she cannot walk.

6. Symptom decreases anxiety and is directly related to the conflict
7. Interventions by nurses
   a. Do not focus on physical symptoms
   b. Minimize sick role behavior
   c. Convey that client is able to perform daily living activities
   d. Identify and reinforce the client's personal strengths
   e. Explore client's relationships with significant others
   f. Explore client's feelings and conflicts
   g. Help client identify what needs are met by symptoms
   h. Help client identify other ways to meet needs

C. Hypochondriasis
   1. Preoccupation with fear of illness or belief that one has an illness based on physical signs
   2. No evidence of illness on physical exam
   3. Symptoms do not result from panic attack
   4. Interventions by nurses
      a. Explore with client the needs being met by symptoms
         (1) Dependency
         (2) Control
         (3) Affection
         (4) Belonging
      b. Explore with client alternative ways of meeting needs without manipulation
      c. Explore client's feelings and conflicts
      d. Help client relate feelings and conflicts to physical symptoms
      e. Do not reinforce sick role

IV. Dissociative disorders

A. A disruption in integrative functions of identity, memory, or consciousness
B. May be transient or well established
C. Associated with exposure to a traumatic event
D. Sexual abuse in childhood is common cause
E. Dissociative identity disorder—multiple personality disorder
   1. Two or more fully developed distinct personalities within an individual
   2. Use of dissociation as a way of distancing and defending self against traumatic experiences and anxiety
   3. Each personality is unique
   4. Transition from one personality to next is sudden and related to stress

     5. Observable personalities in verbal and nonverbal behavior

     6. Personalities may or may not be aware of each other

     7. Each personality represents the individual at different stages of development

     8. Personalities differ in ability to function

     9. Client goal—integration of personalities

F. **Dissociative amnesia**

     1. Unable to recall important personal information because it is anxiety provoking

     2. No organic reason

     3. May deny that gaps in memory exist

     4. Types

        a. Localized—block out all memories about a specified period. Example: car accident.

        b. Selective—recall some but not all memories about a specific period

        c. Generalized—loss of all memory about past life

G. **Dissociative fugue**

     1. Sudden trip away from home or work and the assumption of a new identity

     2. May drift from place to place

     3. Few social relationships during the fugue

     4. When fugue has lifted, client returns home and is unable to remember fugue state (Haber, McMahon, Price-Hoskins, Sideleau, 1992) (see Table 7-2 for diagnosis and statistical profile of various disorders)

H. **Treatment modalities for dissociative disorders**

     1. Individual psychotherapy

     2. Group psychotherapy

     3. Family psychotherapy

I. **Treatment goals for dissociative disorders**

     1. Expanded self-awareness

     2. Integration of dissociated aspects of personality or memory

     3. Increased comfort with self

     4. Decreased anxiety

     5. Increased self-esteem

Table 7-2. Diagnosis and Statistical Profile of Various Disorders

Diagnosis	Statistical Profile
Generalized anxiety disorder	Most frequently found in the general population, equally among both sexes
Panic disorder	Common and equally distributed among men and women; estimated that 2% of population debilitated by disorder; estimated that 4 million Americans suffer from this disorder
Panic disorder with agoraphobia	More common than panic disorder; more common among women
Public disorder	Low frequency of symptoms sufficiently severe to require hospitalization; social and simple phobias relatively common; conflicting data about whether they occur more frequently among men than women; social phobia more common among women; prevalence is higher for blacks than whites, even when demographic and socioeconomic factors are considered
Obsessive-compulsive disorder	Mild forms are common; found equally among men and women; rarely are symptoms sufficiently severe to require hospitalization; estimated that as many as 5 million Americans affected
Somatoform disorder	More common in women; tends to run in families; found less frequently among educated people; associated with alcoholism and sociopathy in male relatives
Conversion disorder	Appears to be less common than 40 or more years ago; seen on neurologic and orthopedic units; increased frequency during war and in military hospitals

Continued.

Table 7-2. Diagnosis and Statistical Profile of Various Disorders—cont'd

Diagnosis	Statistical Profile
Hypochondriasis	Seen by physicians in private practice; found equally among men and women
Dissociative identity disorder	97% of people with this disorder were severely physically and sexually abused and neglected as children; found more frequently among women; probability that it is underdiagnosed in men; men multiples act out violently and may be overrepresented in penal population; occurs in 1.2% of psychiatric population; not as rare as had been thought; increased frequency of assignment of diagnosis
Dissociative amnesia	Rare; increased incidence during war and after natural and technological disasters
Dissociative fugue	Rare; increased incidence during war and after natural and technological disasters; found more frequently among adolescents and young women

Modified from Haber et al: *Comprehensive psychiatric nursing,* ed 4, 1992, Mosby.

REVIEW QUESTIONS

1. The type of therapy using a machine to assist in reducing anxiety and modifying behavioral responses is
   a. Systematic desensitization
   b. Biofeedback
   c. Aversion
   d. Flooding

2. The night before a final exam a student states, "I'm restless, I can't relax, and I want to walk." This individual is at what level of anxiety?
   a. Level I, mild anxiety
   b. Level II, moderate anxiety
   c. Level III, severe anxiety
   d. Level IV, panic

3. Secondary gains or support from others obtained from being sick is characteristic of
   a. Conversion disorders
   b. Anxiety disorders
   c. Bipolar disorders
   d. Dissociative disorders

4. The situation in which individuals have excessive worry or belief that they are suffering from a physical illness despite lack of medical evidence is known as
   a. Psychogenic pain
   b. Psychogenic fugue
   c. Hypochondriasis
   d. Conversion disorder

5. The term "la belle indifference" can best be described as
   a. Longstanding feelings of inferiority
   b. Situations that threaten self-esteem
   c. Marked lack of subjective distress toward symptoms
   d. Partially expressed forbidden impulses

6. A disorder where an individual may manifest a personality that is opposite to a previous identity is
   a. Psychogenic amnesia
   b. Somatoform disorder
   c. La belle indifference
   d. Psychogenic fugue

ANSWERS, RATIONALES, AND TEST-TAKING TIPS

Rationales	Test-Taking Tips

1. Correct answer: b

Biofeedback provides an individual with visual or auditory information about the autonomic physiologic functions of his/her body using instruments. With repeated sessions, the individual learns to control these functions (i.e., blood pressure, pulse, and respirations). This method is used to treat conditions such as hypertension, insomnia, and migraine headaches. Systematic desensitization is a technique of behavior therapy that involves the pairing of deep muscle relaxation with imagined scenes depicting situations that cause the client to feel anxious. Aversion, a behavioral approach, is the initiation of a painful stimulus to create an aversion to another stimulus, which leads to a desired behavior. Flooding is the use of real or imaginary situations to evoke strong anxiety responses.

Think of machines being used in many aspects of medicine to give feedback, such as ECG and CT scan. Thus make an educated guess to select option *b*, biofeedback. Tell yourself, "I know something; I'll figure it out!"

2. Correct answer: a

During this level the individual experiences moderate to low tension but continues to remain in control. The perceptual field is increased, and increased learning may

Use logic to choose option *a*. The information in the stem is generalized with the indication that the student is still in control, so the level of anxiety is most likely the lowest level, mild.

take place. In moderate anxiety the person has a narrowed perceptual field. In severe anxiety the person has a greatly reduced perceptual field and needs direction to focus. At the panic level the person is unable to do things, even with direction.

3. **Correct answer: a**

In conversion disorders, repressed emotional conflicts are converted into sensory, motor, or visual symptoms. These symptoms have no underlying organic cause and serve to reduce the anxiety. Factors include a desire to avoid unpleasant situations or to obtain sympathy or secondary gains from others. In a general anxiety disorder, the cause can usually be identified. Dissociative disorders are disruptions in the integrative functions of identity, memory, or consciousness from a severely damaging situation such as sexual abuse in childhood.

Recall tips: in *conversion* disorders emotions *convert* into physical findings; in *dissociative* disorders there is *disruption* of mental functioning from a *damaging* past experience; and in *general anxiety* disorders the client *gets answer* for cause of the anxiety.

4. **Correct answer: c**

Hypochondriasis, a type of somatoform disorder, is a chronic, exaggerated concern over physical health not based on any real organic disorders. Characterized by anxiety, depression, and an

Eliminate option *a,* since it is too specific; the information in the stem presents the theme of "physical illness." Option *b* is an incorrect term; it should read "dissociative fugue." Be cautious not to select this as an answer just

unrealistic perception of real or imagined physical symptoms, it is caused by unresolved intrapsychic conflicts and is not related to a conscious decision. Unlike conversion disorder, no actual loss or distortion of function occurs.

because you may not know what it is. Remember to go *with what you know!* In deciding between options *c* and *d,* note that the information gives no clue to any type of conversion of beliefs to physical findings, so select option *c* and not *d,* the conversion disorder.

5. Correct answer: c

La belle indifference is defined as a lack of concern shown by some clients toward physical symptoms. The physical symptoms may relieve anxiety, resulting in an inability to perform an activity, and in secondary gains in the form of manipulation of others, freedom from responsibilities, or economic gain. It classically is found in conversion disorders.

The key word in the stem is "indifference." The only answer that suggests an association with this theme is *c.*

6. Correct answer: d

A psychogenic fugue, also called dissociative fugue, is different from amnesia. The fugue state is characterized by a sudden unexplained trip away from home or work and assumption of a new identity that may or may not differ from original personality traits. When the fugue lifts, the individual may return home and be unable to recall memories of the experiences. Psychogenic amnesia, also

Recall tips. Somatoform disorders have symptoms of physical findings associated with anxiety. *La belle indifference* is indifference to loss of sensory, motor, or visceral bodily functions. Amnesia is absence of memory to varying degrees for anxiety. Fugue can be thought of as a fugitive state where a new identity is acted out in a new location.

called dissociative amnesia, is an inability to recall important personal information because it may be anxiety provoking. Somatoform disorders are conversion reactions and hypochondriasis. *La belle indifference* is defined as a lack of concern shown by some clients toward physical symptoms.

Psychosexual Disorders

STUDY OUTCOMES

After completing this chapter, the reader will be able to do the following:

▼ Discuss the role of the nurse as it relates to human sexuality.

▼ Apply the nursing process to clients with psychosexual disorders.

▼ Describe client behaviors associated with psychosexual disorders.

▼ Discuss myths related to human sexuality and psychosexual disorders.

▼ Analyze own feelings and responses to clients with psychosexual disorders.

KEY TERM

Sexuality | One's sense of being a sexual individual; includes how one looks, behaves, and relates to others.

CONTENT REVIEW

I. Self-awareness of the nurse as related to human sexuality (Figure 8-1)
A. Explore one's own feelings and values
   1. Social
   2. Cultural
   3. Familial
B. Feelings related to sexuality
   1. Anxiety
      a. Beliefs and values cause internal conflict
      b. May fail to hear what client is saying
   2. Anger
      a. Toward peers for their values
      b. Toward clients. Examples: abortion, homosexuality.
      c. Toward perpetrators. Example: rape.

II. Predisposing factors for psychosexual disorders
A. Psychoanalytic view
   1. Sexuality formed early in life
   2. Central to personality development
   3. Instinctual drive (libido) necessary for life
B. Biological view
   1. Physical characteristics
   2. Genetics
      a. XX chromosomes female
      b. XY chromosomes male
C. Behavioral view
   1. Physiological components
   2. Psychological components
   3. Learned stimulus

III. Modes of sexual expression
A. Heterosexuality
   1. Male/female sexual relationships
   2. Most common sexual expression

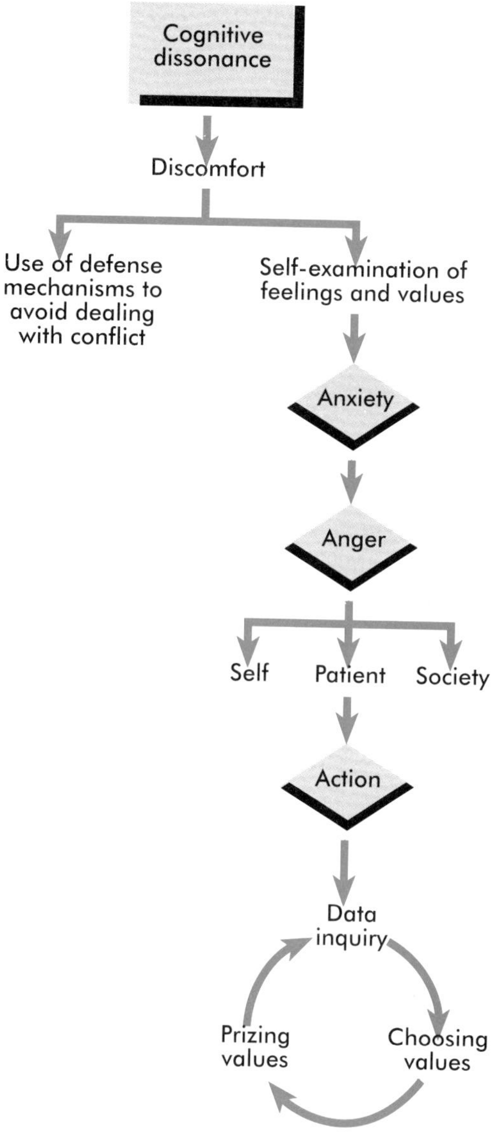

Figure 8-1. Phase in the nurse's growth in developing self-awareness of human sexuality. (From Stuart G and Sundeen S: *Principles and practice of psychiatric nursing,* ed 5, St Louis, 1995, Mosby.)

B. Homosexuality
1. Sexual attraction to member of the same sex
2. Usually act on these feelings
3. Historically, has been considered a maladaptive state
4. Today viewed as sexual expression

      5. Function as well as heterosexuals
        a. Psychologically
        b. Emotionally
        c. Sexually (Stuart and Sundeen, 1991)

  C. Bisexuality
      1. Sexual attraction to and activity with both sexes
      2. May prefer one gender over another
      3. May have one partner or many

  D. Transvestism
      1. Cross-dressing
      2. Obsession with clothing of opposite sex
      3. Usually occurs in married, heterosexual men

IV. Psychosexual disorders

  A. Transsexualism
      1. Feeling that one's assigned sex is inappropriate
      2. Wish to eliminate one's sexual characteristics and acquire those of the opposite sex
      3. Person has reached puberty

  B. Exhibitionism
      1. Recurrent sexual urges and fantasies
      2. Exposure of one's genitals to stranger

  C. Fetishism
      1. Intense sexual images and fantasies
      2. Involves the use of nonliving objects for sexual gratification
        a. Underwear
        b. Socks
        c. Shoes

  D. Pedophilia
      1. Sexual activity with child under age 13
      2. Individual is older than 16 and at least 5 years older than child

  E. Sexual masochism: sexual gratification that involves receiving pain
      1. Humiliation
      2. Beating
      3. Bondage

  F. Sexual sadism: sexual gratification that involves inflicting pain
      1. Psychological suffering
      2. Physical suffering

  G. Voyeurism—receiving sexual gratification through observing others disrobing or engaging in sexual activity

H. **Hypoactive sexual desire**
   1. Lack of desire for sexual activity
   2. Need to assess age, sex, health, and interpersonal relationships
I. **Sexual arousal disorder**
   1. Female—failure to attain or maintain lubrication; swelling is a response to sexual activity
   2. Male—partial or complete failure to attain erection or maintain it until completion of sexual activity
J. **Inhibited orgasm**
   1. Female—persistent or recurrent delay in or absence of orgasm; in some females orgasm only possible with clitoral stimulation
   2. Males—delay in or absence of ejaculation following sexual excitement
K. **Premature ejaculation**
   1. Ejaculation occurs with minimal sexual stimulation
   2. Occurs shortly after penetration
   3. Occurs before individual desires it
L. **Dyspareunia—genital pain before, during, or after sexual intercourse**
M. **Vaginismus**
   1. Involuntary muscle spasm in outer third of the vagina that interferes with coitus
   2. Not exclusively a physical problem

V. Application of the nursing process

A. **Assessment**
   1. Sexual history should be discussed
   2. Open-ended questions
      a. How would you describe your current sexual activity?
      b. Do you have any health problems that affect your sexual activity?
      c. Are you taking any medications that affect your sexual activity?
      d. What, if anything, would you change about your current sexual activity? (Stuart and Sundeen, 1991)
   3. Precipitating events for sexual disorders
      a. Physical illness
         (1) Change in body image
         (2) Decrease in libido
         (3) Fear. Example: clients with cardiac problems.

           (4) Spinal cord injuries

           (5) Diabetes

       b. Medications

           (1) Impotence

           (2) Failure to ejaculate

           (3) Orgasmic dysfunctions

       c. Fear of sexually transmitted diseases

       d. Aging

           (1) Myth of disinterest

           (2) Described as oversexed or "dirty old men"/"dirty old women"

    4. Do not push client to discuss sexual issues—refer to later

  B. Interventions

    1. Primary prevention

       a. Education

       b. All sexual thoughts are normal

       c. Sexuality is part of identity

    2. Secondary prevention (Table 8-1, 8-2)

Table 8-1. Plan of Care—Clients with Sexual Dysfunction

Long-term Outcomes	Short-term Outcomes	Nursing Strategies
Nursing diagnosis: Sexual dysfunction secondary to inability to achieve a satisfactory ejaculatory response related to values conflict with partner (NANDA 3.2.1.2.1; DSM-III-R 302.75)		
Experience satisfying ejaculatory response within the context of the relationship with a partner to explore personal value systems as it relates to sexual behavior	To establish working relationship with nurse To develop more effective communication skills with partner To participate in sensate focus exercises with partner To utilize "stop-start" or "squeeze" technique	Provide an atmosphere that permits clients to be sexual Complete a detailed sexual history Discuss the need for accountability to perform exercises Follow process for "stop-start" or "squeeze" technique Discuss potential and actual problems encountered with therapy Identify current stressors that may be related to personal value system Describe measures for mediating stressors

Table 8-2. **Plan of Care—Clients with Sexual Dysfunction**

Long-term Outcomes	Short-term Outcomes	Nursing Strategies
Nursing diagnosis: Increased anxiety related to fear of public awareness of homosexual orientation (NANDA 9.3.1; DSM-III-R 302.0)		
Develop a positive sense of self as a sexual being Demonstrate a decreased anxiety level	Identify precipitators of anxiety Explore personal value system regarding homosexuality Discuss myths regarding homosexuals and their lifestyle	Demonstrate acceptance of choice of homosexual orientation Suggest specific literature on homosexuality to increase knowledge base Encourage exploration of personal beliefs regarding homosexual behavior Discuss client's perceptions of cause of anxiety Explore methods to reduce anxiety Test out strategies through role play Encourage use of support groups for homosexuals and lesbians

3. Tertiary
   a. Psychoanalysis
   b. Individual and couples therapy
C. Evaluation—client has
   1. A reduction in anxiety
   2. An increase in sexual satisfaction
   3. A decrease in ejaculatory incompetence
   4. Used referrals to other health professionals, such as sex therapists
   5. Used referrals to community resources
      a. Attended support groups for gays and lesbians, if appropriate
      b. Attended support groups for people with chronic illnesses, if indicated

REVIEW QUESTIONS

1. A college student enters the health clinic in a hysterical state, exclaiming that two people riding the elevator exposed their genitals by lifting their skirts between floors. The nurse identifies this behavior as
   a. Sexual sadism
   b. Exhibitionism
   c. Fetishism
   d. Transsexualism

2. After initial assessment of the client with a psychosexual disorder, the nurse would more commonly
   a. Initiate therapy
   b. Refer the client to the appropriate therapist
   c. Refer the client to the appropriate support group
   d. Test out new coping strategies through role play

3. On a routine exam the client complains of dysparenunia. The nurse would obtain further information about this problem. Which statement would the nurse most likely make next?
   a. "Tell me more about this pain with the act of sexual intercourse"
   b. "Tell me more about your inability to have an orgasm"
   c. "What if anything has changed about your sex drive?"
   d. "Are you taking any medications that affect your sexual arousal?"

ANSWERS, RATIONALES, AND TEST-TAKING TIPS

Rationales	Test-Taking Tips

1. Correct answer: b

Exhibitionism is the exposure of one's genitals to strangers. Sexual sadism is sexual gratification that involves inflicting psychological or physical pain or suffering. Fetishism is intense sexual images and fantasies that involve the use on nonliving objects for sexual gratification such as shoes or underwear. Transsexualism is feeling that one's assigned sex is inappropriate with the wish to eliminate one's sexual characteristics and acquire those of the opposite sex.

If you have no idea of the correct answer, simply match the behavior of the strangers, they exhibited themselves, and select option *b* that has this word in it.

2. Correct answer: b

The nurse would more commonly refer the client to a therapist for individual therapy. Nurses would initiate therapy only if they had advanced degrees and specialized in this area. Support group referral would be at a later time. Testing out new strategies is inappropriate at this time.

The key words in the stem are "after the initial assessment" and "more commonly." If nurses are not specialists in the area specified then the more common action is to refer to qualified professionals.

3. Correct answer: a

Dyspareunia is the occurrence of genital pain either before, during or after sexual intercourse. The other options are incorrect.

On this type of question if you have no idea of the correct answer, simply narrow the responses to either options *a* or *b* that begin with "tell me . . ." which is a broad opening. From here make your best educated guess, take a few deep breaths, and go on to the next question. Remember that there will be questions on the exam you have no idea of the correct answer. Avoid letting these type of questions make you too tense or tired to think clearly on the questions that you know.

Personality Disorders

STUDY OUTCOMES

After completing this chapter, the reader will be able to do
the following:

▼ Describe behaviors exhibited by a client with the medical diagnosis
of a personality disorder.

▼ Discuss the theories on the causes of personality disorders.

▼ Discuss symptoms of the various diagnostic categories of the
DSM IV.

▼ List examples of nursing diagnoses applicable to clients
experiencing various personality disorders.

▼ Apply the nursing process with clients experiencing various
personality disorders.

KEY TERMS

Impaired impulse control	Impulsivity and feelings of emptiness, boredom, and rage cause physical assaults on environment, others, and themselves (Taylor, 1994).
Manipulation	Process of influencing another to meet one's own needs and desires, regardless of the needs and desires of another (Rawlins et al, 1993).
Mood	A prolonged emotional state that influences one's whole personality and life functioning (Stuart and Sundeen, 1991).
Object relations	Degree and quality of relatedness to others (Haber, et al, 1992).
Personality traits	Characteristics of individuals that make them unique and form the basis for how they perceive the world and relate to others (Taylor, 1994).
Separation-individualization process	Development of a unified sense of self in which the personality is integrated (Taylor, 1994).
Splitting	Viewing people and situations as either all good or all bad; failure to integrate the positive and negative qualities of oneself (Stuart and Sundeen, 1991).

CONTENT REVIEW

I. Personality Disorders

A. Lifelong patterns of maladaptive behavior
B. Three clusters of personality disorders (Box 9-1)
C. Not based on sound personality structure
D. Difficult to change
E. Not distressing to person with the personality disorder
F. Common character traits in individuals with a personality disorder
   1. Poor impulse control
      a. Uncontrollable pressure to act on internal urges
      b. Act out to manage internal pain
      c. Little reflection in introspection
      d. Forms of acting-out behavior
         (1) Physical attacks
         (2) Verbal attacks

Box 9-1. Clusters of Personality Disorders

Cluster 1—Eccentric

Paranoid: suspicious, quarrelsome, relies excessively on projection
Schizoid: lethargic, unresponsive, relies excessively on intellectualization
Schizotypal: eccentric, isolative, relies excessively on undoing

Cluster 2—Erratic

Histrionic: dramatic, demanding, relies excessively on dissociation
Narcissistic: arrogant, exploitive, fragile, relies excessively on rationalization
Antisocial: impulsive, irresponsible, relies excessively on acting out
Borderline: impulsive, conflicted, relies excessively on regression

Cluster 3—Fearful

Avoidant: guarded, private, relies excessively on fantasy
Dependent: incompetent, helpless, relies excessively on introjection
Compulsive: perfectionistic, driven, relies excessively on reaction formation
Passive-aggressive: competitive, intimidating, relies excessively on reaction
    formation

From Haber J, et al: *Comprehensive psychiatric nursing,* ed 4, St Louis, 1992, Mosby.

      (3) Manipulation
      (4) Abuse of substances
      (5) Promiscuous sexual behaviors with any available person and often with animals
      (6) Suicide attempts
2. Mood characteristics—abandonment depression: when significant people in their lives are absent they feel abandoned
   a. Painful, dysphonic feelings
   b. Rage
   c. Guilt
   d. Fear
   e. Emptiness
3. Impaired judgment in individuals experiencing a personality disorder
   a. Have impaired problem-solving abilities
   b. Do not perceive consequences of behaviors
   c. Do not learn from past behaviors

    4. Impaired reality testing in individuals experiencing a personality disorder
      a. Distort inner and outer reality
      b. Often project their own feelings onto others. Example: think another person is angry toward themselves.
    5. Impaired object relations in individuals experiencing a personality disorder
      a. Difficulty in intimate relationships
      b. Rigid and inflexible way of relating
    6. Impaired perception of self in individuals experiencing a personality disorder
      a. Distorted perception of self
      b. Self-hate or self-idealization
    7. Impaired thought process in individuals experiencing a personality disorder
      a. Impaired thinking
        (1) Concrete
        (2) Diffuse
      b. Impaired concentration
      c. Impaired memory
    8. Impaired stimulus barrier (inability to regulate incoming sensory stimuli as it occurs) in individuals experiencing a personality disorder
      a. Increased excitability—feel like "jumping out of skin"
      b. Excessive response to noise and light
      c. Behaviors
        (1) Agitation
        (2) Insomnia
        (3) Poor attention

G. Theories of causality of personality disorders
    1. No theory of mental illness is proven
    2. Ego development
      a. Normal development
        (1) Infant begins at around 6 months to perceive that mother and self are separate
        (2) Splitting normally occurs—pleasure from "good" mom, pain from "bad" mom
        (3) Normal splitting preserves relationship with mom
        (4) Next stage is integration of good-bad, love-hate

      b. Personality disorder—mothering one responds to child in a way that causes frustration or physical and/or emotional pain

          (1) Unrelenting frustration or pain—aggression toward "bad mother"; pathological splitting continues to defend against aggression

          (2) Lack of integration of aggression and love

   3. Separation-individuation

      a. Normal development

          (1) 18 months to 3 years

          (2) Parallels physical separation from mom through walking

          (3) Object constancy—ability to evoke a stable and consistent mental image of mother in her absence

      b. Personality disorder—does not obtain object constancy; separation not supported by mother, as mother withdraws love during behaviors of individuation; fear of abandonment and separation from others means total loss of connection

H. Ten types of personality disorders found in the DSM-IV

   1. Schizoid personality disorder

      a. Social detachment

      b. Restricted expression of emotions

      c. Lack of close relationships

      d. Aloofness

      e. Indifference

      f. Interest in solitary activities

      g. Little interest in sexual experiences

      h. Lack of interest in others' responses or feelings

      i. "Drift" with goals

   2. Schizotypal personality disorder

      a. Relationship deficits

      b. Suspiciousness

      c. Paranoid ideation

      d. Magical thinking

      e. Unusual perceptual experiences

      f. Odd thinking and speech

   3. Paranoid personality disorder

      a. Distrust

      b. Suspiciousness

      c. Others' motives interpreted as malevolent

      d. Argumentative

      e. Hostile aloofness

      f. Appears cold and lacking in tender feeling

      g. Rigid

      h. Critical of others

      i. Controlling of others

      j. Grandiosity—a sense of self-importance or of entitlement to special treatment

4. Histrionic personality disorder

      a. Emotionality

      b. Attention-seeking behavior

      c. Needs to be center of attention

      d. Sexually provocative or seductive

      e. Overly concerned with appearance

      f. Theatrical

      g. Self-dramatizing

      h. Has romantic fantasies

      i. Controls partners

      j. Bored easily

      k. Dependency

5. Narcissistic personality disorder

      a. Grandiosity—a sense of self-importance or entitlement to special treatment

      b. Needs admiration

      c. Lacks empathy

      d. Overestimates abilities

      e. Inflates accomplishments

      f. Underestimates contributions of others

      g. Fragile self-esteem

      h. Lacks sensitivity to needs and wants of others

6. Avoidant personality disorder

      a. Social inhibition

      b. Feelings of inadequacy

      c. Hypersensitive to reactions of others

      d. Reacts poorly to criticism

      e. Small support system

      f. Avoidance of social situations impairs upward mobility in jobs

      g. Avoids people unless certain to be liked

7. Dependent personality disorder

      a. Difficulty making decisions

      b. Needs others to assume responsibility for activities of daily living

      c. Cannot disagree with others

    d. Refrains from independent actions—lacks autonomy

    e. Cannot tolerate being alone

    f. Must always have a close relationship

    g. Fears being left to care for self

8. Obsessive-compulsive personality disorder

    a. Orderliness

    b. Perfectionism

    c. Mental and interpersonal control

    d. Preoccupied with rules and details

    e. Devoted to work and productivity

    f. Lacks leisure activities and friendships

    g. Overconscientious

    h. Inflexible

    i. Reluctant to delegate tasks

    j. Miserly

    k. Stubborn

    l. Hoards worthless objects

9. Antisocial personality disorder

    a. History

        (1) Long history of dysfunctional interpersonal relationships and occupational endeavors

        (2) Criminal record

        (3) Dependence on alcohol or drugs

        (4) Sexually deviant behavior

        (5) Absence of guilt or remorse

        (6) Rationalizes or justifies behavior

    b. Behavior characteristics

        (1) Ability to be charming

        (2) Unable to tolerate frustration

        (3) Want what they want when they want it

        (4) Views others as objects to be manipulated

        (5) Poor judgment and insight

        (6) Does not learn from experience

        (7) Lack of responsibility

        (8) Impulsivity

10. Borderline personality disorder (Clinical Example 9-1)

    a. May be a precursor to a dissociative disorder, such as a multiple personality disorder

    b. Lacks integrated sense of self—unclear identity, including sexual identity, as well as lack of awareness of strengths and weaknesses

Clinical Example 9-1. Borderline Personality Disorder

The client is a 30-year-old, single white female with a history of 40 inpatient psychiatric admissions over the last 10 years. She has scar tissue extending from her wrists to her elbows on both arms, with a visual absence of normal tissue. This scar tissue has been caused by repeated, self-inflicted razor blade cuts. The client explains that she cuts herself to "feel good" when she is experiencing emotional distress in her life. The kinds of emotional distress that have caused this behavior in the past are as follows: a fight with her mother, her therapist's being on vacation, and the breakup of a relationship. She describes feeling abandoned in these situations, and says the only thing that helps her to feel better is the physical act of cutting. The client describes the cutting and bleeding process as an emotional catharsis.

     c. Fear of being alone
     d. Splitting—all things, including self, are all good or all bad
     e. Relationships characterized by "yo yo" syndrome—approach/avoidance
     f. Interpersonal closeness equals fusion, loss of self
     g. Separation, distance equals abandonment
     h. Extreme shifts in mood
     i. Depression
     j. Anger—particularly related to abandonment issues
     k. Self-destructive behavior
        (1) Cutting—converts emotional pain to physical pain; creates pleasure
        (2) Burning self
        (3) Substance abuse
        (4) Binging
        (5) Suicidal gestures
     l. Manipulation
     m. Lack of object constance—when people are away it feels as if they will never return
     n. Fighting with others
     o. Boredom
     p. Emptiness

  I. Incidence of personality disorders
    1. 5% to 15% of adult population
    2. High incidence in prisons and urban areas
  J. Treatment—psychotherapy (focus)
    1. Ownership of feelings and responsibility
    2. Address abandonment issues

      3. Integration of self-concept

      4. Decrease of splitting as a defense

K. Prognosis

      1. Has historically been considered poor, due to lack of desire for change and longstanding behavioral patterns

      2. Progress is slow

      3. Compliance with treatment is low

      4. New social theories support that personality disorders are dynamic and can be influenced with social support from a stable system

L. Nursing process

      1. Common nursing diagnoses and outcomes (Table 9-1)

      2. Nursing interventions

         a. Inform client that harm to self, others, and property is unacceptable

         b. Receive a written contract from client to follow a plan of care

         c. Help client discuss feelings rather than act them out

         d. Reinforce consistency in staff response to client's acting-out behaviors

         e. Review policies, expectations, and responsibilities to client

         f. Discuss what consequences will follow certain behaviors. Example: acting-out behaviors result in no passes for 48 hours.

         g. Identify splitting behavior—which staff are labeled as "good" and which as "bad"

         h. Point out discrepancies in client's perceptions of staff. Example: one day you are good, the next day bad.

         i. Help client deal directly with anger

         j. All staff should meet as a group with the client to clarify expectations of each person

         k. Hold staff meetings to discuss the process and feelings related to the splitting process

         l. Encourage client to keep a journal that records daily feelings

         m. Maintain safety against self-destructive behaviors

Table 9-1. Nursing Diagnoses and Long-Term Outcomes for Clients with Personality Disorders

Nursing Diagnoses	Client Outcomes
	Client will:
Ineffective individual coping related to fear of abandonment by significant others	Demonstrate knowledge that healthy, mature behavior does not lead to abandonment by significant others
Risk for violence directed at others related to inability to tolerate emotional pain	Verbally express feelings rather than act out
Risk for violence: self-directed related to defense against abandonment depression	Express discomfort with self-destructive behavior
Ineffective individual coping related to the splitting mechanism	Describe others as having both good and bad qualities
Risk for violence: self-directed related to activation of abandonment depression	Verbalize and rechannel feelings of depression
Risk for violence: directed at others related to excessive aggression and poor impulse control	Refrain from hurting self and others
Self-esteem disturbance related to clinging, regressive, lifeless behavior	Establish healthy relationship with one authority figure
Noncompliance with milieu structure related to self-concept of being special and exempt from rules and expectations	Hold self accountable for consequences of violation of structure and expectations
A loneliness and emptiness related to conflicts that impede interpersonal closeness and intimacy	Retain a consistent degree of relatedness with selected others in spite of emotional conflicts and upheaval
Personal identity disturbance related to incomplete separation-individuation from maternal object	Continually clarify own thoughts, goals, values, and feelings with staff
Anxiety related to client's feelings of being reunited with the "good mother" or abandoned by the "bad mother"	Relate fluctuation in moods to internal processes rather than perceiving them as environmentally induced

From Haber J, et al: *Comprehensive psychiatric nursing,* ed 4, St. Louis, 1992, Mosby.

REVIEW QUESTIONS

1. Personality disorders, on the multiaxial diagnosis, appear in
   a. Axis I
   b. Axis II
   c. Axis III
   d. Axis IV

2. A newly admitted client states, "No one cares; everyone is against me." This type of statement is consistent with what disorder?
   a. Paranoid personality disorder
   b. Schizoid personality disorder
   c. Schizotypal personality disorder
   d. Antisocial personality disorder

3. Clients with an antisocial disorder may not profit by psychotherapy because they
   a. Do not have the intelligence to profit from therapy
   b. Have difficulty relating meaningfully
   c. Are too psychotic to cooperate
   d. Will not accept the therapy

4. Your client states, "I work for the government, and I am so important in my office that the other people will not be able to work without me." This is characteristic of
   a. A histrionic personality disorder
   b. An antisocial personality disorder
   c. A narcissistic personality disorder
   d. A multiple personality disorder

5. A client is diagnosed as a borderline personality disorder. An important characteristic displayed in this client is an inability to incorporate all good or all bad. This is known as
   a. Denial
   b. Splitting
   c. Sublimation
   d. Regression

ANSWERS, RATIONALES, AND TEST-TAKING TIPS

Rationales	Test-Taking Tips

1. Correct answer: b

According to the multiaxial diagnosis in the DSM IV, all personality disorders are Axis II diagnoses.

The best approach to this type of question is to take a few deep breaths, reread the question, then make your best educated guess. If you have no idea, it is usually best to eliminate the extremes, then select the most conservative number or level. Refrain from getting emotionally reactive to these types of questions. You must remain calm, refreshed, and objective for the remainder of the examination.

2. Correct answer: a

This disorder is characterized by pervasive and unwarranted suspiciousness and mistrust of others. Individuals with this disorder will not give up the suspiciousness even when presented with convincing evidence to dispute their suspiciousness. Schizoid personality disorder has characteristics of social detachment, restricted expression of emotions, and lack of close relationships. Schizotypal personality disorder has the characteristics of relationship deficits, suspiciousness, magical thinking, and odd thinking and speech. Antisocial personality disorder is associated with histories of

The key words in the stem are "everyone is against me." This is typical of a paranoid personality disorder.

dysfunctional interpersonal relationships and job endeavors, criminal records, and absence of guilt or remorse. The characteristics of antisocial personalities include abilities to be charming, to views others as objects to be manipulated, to not learn from experiences, to lack responsibility, and to act impulsively.

3. Correct answer: b

Because these clients are unstable in mood and self-image, they are not able to sustain interpersonal relationships. They view everyone and everything as all good or all bad and cannot see both qualities. They do not learn from experience, lack insight, and show poor judgment. The other options are incorrect.

These types of clients do have intelligence, are not psychotic, and may typically act to accept therapy, since they have the ability to be charming.

4. Correct answer: c

This condition is characterized by an exaggerated sense of self-importance and uniqueness. This individual has an abnormal need for attention and admiration and usually experiences disturbances in relationships. Histrionic personality disorder includes characteristics of being overly concerned with appearance, needing to be the center of attention, getting bored easily,

Think of narcissistic as an egotistic, self-admiring finding in a personality disorder. The other word to associate is "grandiosity," which implies a sense of self-importance or entitlement to special treatment. The comment in the stem given by the client reflects this personality.

and exhibiting attention-seeking behaviors. Antisocial personality disorder is associated with histories of dysfunctional interpersonal relationships and job endeavors, criminal records, and absence of guilt or remorse. The characteristics of antisocial personalities include abilities to be charming, to view others as objects to be manipulated, to not learn from experiences, to lack responsibility, and to act impulsively. Multiple personality disorder, also called dissociative identity disorder, is a type of dissociative disorder in which there is a disruption in the functions of identity into two or more personalities in order to deal with traumatic experiences.

5. **Correct answer: b**

Splitting is a primitive defense mechanism. There is a failure to recognize the positive and negative experiences one has of himself/herself, other people, and situations. Denial is no acknowledgement of a situation or emotion. Sublimation is acceptance of a socially approved substitute goal for a drive whose normal channel of expression is blocked. Regression is the return to behaviors or thoughts to an earlier level of development.

Use an educated guess to eliminate options *a* and *d.* With the options narrowed to either *b* or *c,* reread the stem carefully and note the key words, "inability to incorporate all good or bad." This seems to describe a splitting. Select option *b.*

Eating Disorders

STUDY OUTCOMES

After completing this chapter, the reader will be able to do the following:

▼ Define compulsive overeating, anorexia nervosa, and bulimia nervosa.
▼ Describe the theoretical bases for eating disorders.
▼ Describe the dysfunctional behaviors of clients experiencing eating disorders.
▼ Apply the nursing process to clients experiencing eating disorders.

KEY TERMS

Anorexia nervosa	Eating disorder of life-threatening proportion, characterized by relentless pursuit of thinness, intense fear of becoming fat, and delusional disturbance of body image (Haber et al, 1992).
Bulimia nervosa or binge-purge syndrome	Episodic, rapid consumption of large amounts of food in a short time; termination of eating episode results from abdominal pain, sleep, social interruption, or self-induced vomiting (Haber et al, 1992).
Compulsive overeating	Food consumption is out of an individual's control and according to fixed rules or in a stereotyped fashion (Haber et al, 1992).
Obesity	Weight 15% to 20% more than one's ideal body weight, with an excessive proportion of fat or adipose tissue in the body mass.

CONTENT REVIEW

I. Eating disorders
   A. Dysfunctional eating behavioral patterns
      1. Overconsumption or underconsumption of food
      2. Linked with one's earliest emotional needs within the context of feeding
      3. Cultural influence of thinness
      4. Cultural preoccupation with the pleasures of eating
      5. Importance of beauty
   B. Compulsive overeating
      1. Binge-like overeating
      2. One in five Americans is obese (weight 15 to 20% more than ideal body weight)
      3. Eating relieves tension but does not produce pleasure
      4. Does not purge
      5. May be repulsed by eating
      6. Lacks interest in exercise programs
      7. Feels helpless and hopeless about weight
      8. Responds by eating when experiencing certain feelings
         a. Guilt
         b. Anger
         c. Boredom
         d. Inadequacy

            e. Ambivalence

            f. Loneliness

      8. Aware that eating patterns are abnormal

      9. Feels depressed after eating

    10. Consumes high-calorie, easily digested food

    11. Eats secretly during binge

    12. Repeatedly tries dieting to lose weight, but without success

    13. Weight fluctuations of greater than 10 pounds caused by alternating binging and dieting

    14. Precipitants to eating

            a. Anger

            b. Depression

            c. Marital conflict in parents

            d. Family traditions or beliefs

            e. Parents with addictive behaviors

    15. No body image disturbance

C. **Anorexia nervosa (Clinical Example 10-1)**

      1. Emotional symptoms

            a. Body image distortion—feels fat even when cachexic

            b. Preoccupation with foods that prevent weight gain

            c. Phobia against foods that produce weight gain

            d. Emaciated appearance

            e. Fear of sexual maturity

            f. Feelings of lack of control

Clinical Example 10-1. Anorexia Nervosa

The client is a 24-year-old, single white female standing 5 feet 2 inches and weighing 65 pounds. She has been in and out of psychiatric inpatient units since age 14. She describes the onset of her eating disorder as an attempt to stop the development of secondary sexual characteristics. Until age 12, she played baseball routinely with her father and various boys in her neighborhood. When the client was 12, her father informed her that she could no longer play with the boys without wearing a shirt, because she was developing breasts. She became concerned that she would no longer be able to play with the boys and with her dad if she continued to develop breasts. At the time of her present admission, she has not eaten solid foods in 2 years and has sustained herself with liquid nutrition such as Ensure. She refuses to eat with other clients and insists on working with a select group of staff. She is suffering from numerous electrolyte imbalances, hypotension, cyanotic extremities, dry, scaly skin, and bradycardia, yet insists that she is fat.

g. Disturbed self-concept

h. Depression

2. Behavioral symptoms

    a. Major reduction in food intake

    b. Self-induced vomiting—may use emetics

    c. Self-administered enemas (several a week to several a day)

    d. Excessive exercise

    e. Overachievement

    f. Perfectionism

3. Physical symptoms (listed most common to least common)

    a. Amenorrhea for at least three consecutive menstrual periods

    b. Hypotension

    c. Electrolyte imbalance

    d. Sleep disturbance

    e. Increased body hair

    f. Scaly skin

    g. Hypothermia

    h. Cyanosis and numbness of extremities

    i. Bradycardia

    j. Gastritis

    k. Teeth and gum deterioration due to effects of hydrochloric acid from the stomach during emesis

    l. Delayed stomach emptying

    m. Estrogen deficiency

    n. Lowered testosterone production

    o. Anemia

    p. Decreased WBCs

    q. Decreased platelet levels

    r. Elevated cholesterol levels

    s. Weakened heart muscle

    t. Decreased cardiac output

    u. Osteoporosis

    v. Peripheral nerve paralysis

    w. Esophageal varices from increased venous pressure during emesis

4. Prevalence and epidemiology (DSM IV, 1994)

    a. In females 0.5 to 1.0% who meet full criteria; individuals who are subthreshold for the disorder are more common

    b. 95% are females

    c. Limited data for males

    d. Incidence has increased in recent decades

      e. Mean age of onset is 17 years

      f. Onset often associated with a stressful life event

      g. Long-term mortality is greater than 10%

      h. Death typically occurs from starvation, suicide, electrolyte imbalance

5. Treatment
   a. Antidepressant medication
   b. Restoration of fluid and electrolyte balance
   c. Assertiveness training
   d. Support groups
   e. Psychotherapy—focuses on
      (1) Control
      (2) Identity
      (3) Independence
      (4) Self-esteem

6. Course of disorder
   a. Some clients recover after single episode
   b. Other clients fluctuate with relapses
   c. Other clients deteriorate over the years and may die

D. Bulimia nervosa

1. Binge-purge syndrome
2. Consumes high-calorie, easily digested food in secret
3. Tries to lose weight through diets, self-induced vomiting, enemas, cathartics, amphetamines, or diuretics
4. Weight fluctuations may be greater than 10 pounds in one day
5. Weight is within normal weight-height parameters
6. Appears physically well
7. Preoccupied with body shape and weight; however, usually no body image distortion
8. Physical complications
   a. Loss of tooth enamel
   b. Dental decay
   c. Receding gums
   d. Stomach ulcers
   e. Electrolyte imbalance
   f. Rectal bleeding
   g. Heart disease
   h. Hypertension
   i. Diabetes
   j. Esophogeal varices
9. Guilt about secretive eating
10. Self-mutilative behaviors

11. Suicidal thoughts
12. Mood swings
13. Suicide attempts
14. Prevalence and epidemiology (DSM IV, 1994)
    a. Not identified as disorder until the 1960s and 1970s
    b. Onset of bulimia is common in adolescence or early adulthood
    c. Statistics regarding mortality are unavailable
    d. 90% are females
    e. 1 to 3% of adolescent and young adult females
15. Treatment
    a. Antidepressant medication
    b. Restoration of fluid and electrolyte balance
    c. Treatment for mood disorder and anxiety disorder
    d. Support groups
    e. Psychotherapy
        (1) Control
        (2) Self-esteem
        (3) Autonomy
        (4) Identity
16. Course of disorder
    a. Binge eating begins related to dieting
    b. Chronic or intermittent occurrence
    c. Eating behavior often persists for several years
E. **Three theories of causality of eating disorders**
    1. Physiologic theory
        a. Theories about nutrients and appetite regulators such as peptides, glucose, fatty acids, amino acids, purines
        b. Hypothalamus disorder—neurotransmitters, hypothalamic secretions
        c. Endocrine disturbances: hypothalamic pituitary—adrenal; hypothalamic pituitary—thyroid
    2. Cognitive-behavioral theory
        a. Learned maladaptive behaviors
        b. Emphasize observable behavioral events and eating responses
        c. Two conflicts
            (1) Avoidance-avoidance, such as avoiding gaining weight and avoiding being ill
            (2) Approach-avoidance; ambivalent feelings to same object. For instance, wants to lose weight but does not want to decrease food intake.

3. Family theory for anorexia
   a. Overprotection by hypervigilant parents
   b. Rigid boundaries
   c. Enmeshed families
   d. Stressful events in families trigger behaviors
   e. Controlling mothers and distant fathers
   f. Go-between role between parents
   g. Involved in spousal conflict
   h. Loyal to family values
   i. Onset of anorexia often linked to
      (1) Loss
      (2) Separation
      (3) Change in family
   j. Family unites to "protect" anorexic child
   k. Weight and food become central family concern
4. Family theory for bulimia (Table 10-1)
   a. Parents often obese

Table 10-1. Family Dynamics of Bulimic Persons

Family Dynamics	Resulting Behaviors
Low level of self-differentiation	Sacrifice of self in an attempt to control the addictive behaviors of other family members Assumption of responsibility for meeting others' needs to the exclusion of one's own Nonconformity as a means of asserting control Deep-rooted shame and guilt Feelings of inadequacy
Enmeshment	Increased anxiety in intimate relationships Fear of abandonment Fear of loss and separation Excessive respect for paternal authority
Cross-generational transmission of anxiety	One or more close family members who are alcoholic Presence of physical or sexual abuse Learned patterns of avoidant behavior in response to stress

Haber J, et al: *Comprehensive psychiatric nursing*, ed 4, St Louis, 1992, Mosby.

     b. Chronic illness present in family

     c. Presence of obsessive-compulsive disorders

     d. Phobias

     e. Divorce

     f. Death

     g. High levels of family conflict and marital dissatisfaction (Modified from Haber et al, 1992)

F. **Application of the nursing process for eating disorders**

  1. Assessment

     a. History of eating problem

        (1) What is current height and weight?

        (2) How does your current height and weight vary from ideal?

        (3) What were highest and lowest weights and when did they occur?

        (4) What were past eating patterns like before the eating disorder?

        (5) What was happening in your life just before the onset of the eating disorder?

        (6) How long ago did the binge and purge episodes begin?

        (7) How many binge and purge cycles occur in a week?

        (8) Is there a pattern to the binge and purge cycles?

     b. Other areas of assessment

        (1) How often do you think about food in a 24-hour period?

        (2) Do you ever eat in secret?

        (3) Do you ever cause yourself to vomit?

        (4) Do you ever take laxatives or diuretics?

           (a) How often?

           (b) What type?

           (c) What dosage?

        (5) Do you ever take amphetamines or over-the-counter stimulants?

        (6) Describe the frequency and the type of your exercise

        (7) Do you feel fat or thin?

        (8) Draw a picture of yourself

        (9) Do you experience amenorrhea or irregular menses?

        (10) Do you eat at night?

        (11) Do you binge at night?

        (12) Is there a history of sexual abuse?

        (13) Are you sexually active?

        (14) Describe a typical family mealtime

        (15) Which of your family members are overweight? Too thin?

        (16) Does anyone in your family eat too much? Too little? (Modified from Haber et al, 1992)

2. Nursing diagnoses for eating disorders
   a. Alteration in nutrition (less than body requirements)
   b. Alteration in nutrition (more than body requirements)
   c. Ineffective individual coping
   d. Alteration in body image
   e. Alteration in mood
   f. Social isolation related to compulsive overeating or misperception of body size

3. Nursing interventions
   a. Group
      (1) Decrease client isolation
      (2) Use peer pressure to change dysfunctional eating patterns
      (3) Change client's self-perceptions through feedback from others
      (4) Refer client to an eating support group
   b. Family
      (1) Psychoeducation
      (2) Cognitive insight
      (3) Adaptive coping
   c. Substitution
      (1) Log eating activities
      (2) Describe feelings, thoughts, stress, boredom, and relationship to eating
      (3) Plan alternative responses
   d. Contracting
      (1) Set of rules and consequences agreed upon by nurse and client
      (2) Differentiate client's motivations from expectations of others
   e. Cognitive restructuring—explore eating beliefs and substitute more healthy ones
   f. Positive and negative reinforcement
   g. Visualization and guided imagery
   h. Assertiveness training
      (1) Link between eating disorders and assertiveness
      (2) Teach client behaviors for giving and accepting compliments
      (3) Teach client behaviors for giving and accepting criticism

REVIEW QUESTIONS

1. Which documentation by the staff indicates that the client has anorexia nervosa?
   a. Outgoing, active, friendly
   b. Diarrhea, fever, increased thirst
   c. Preoccupation with food, disturbed body image, fear of sexual maturity
   d. Preoccupied with body shape, suicidal thoughts, overactivity

2. To assess the eating pattern of a client diagnosed with anorexia nervosa, the nurse might ask the following
   a. "How do you feel about your present weight?"
   b. "Who plans the meals in your family?"
   c. "Do you see yourself as fat?"
   d. "Tell me what you eat in a typical day"

3. A female client has gone from 110 pounds to 90 pounds, and she has stopped menstruating. Based on this information, the nursing diagnosis would be *alteration in nutrition: less then body requirements related to*
   a. Excessive exercise program
   b. Self-induced vomiting
   c. Loss of 15% of body weight
   d. Abuse of laxatives

4. Which statement is true concerning bulimia nervosa?
   a. The age of onset is younger than that of a person with anorexia nervosa
   b. About 40% of bulimics are actually overweight before the onset of the illness
   c. There is an intense fear of foods that produce weight gain
   d. This is an exclusively female disorder

5. In the written assessment of a client with anorexia nervosa, which finding would be least commonly noted?
   a. Amenorrhea
   b. Anemia
   c. Hypotension
   d. Lanugo

ANSWERS, RATIONALES, AND TEST-TAKING TIPS

Rationales	Test-Taking Tips

1. Correct answer: c

The other options are not findings of anorexia nervosa. Preoccupation with body shape and suicidal thoughts are findings in bulema nervosa.

Recall tip: the client with anorexia nervosa has the disturbed body image. If you can only recall this fact, then on this question, go with what you know, and select option *c*.

2. Correct answer: d

Options *a* and *c* focus on feelings and thoughts rather than on diet. Option *b* is irrelevant, since who fixes the food has nothing to do with the anorexic's eating habits.

Note the key words in the stem, "to assess . . . eating patterns." The only option that addresses that focus is *d*.

3. Correct answer: c

The history of the client supports the etiology of this statement for the nursing diagnosis. There is no other information given to support the remaining three options.

The approach to this question is to make your selection, then reread the question with your chosen answer to make sure you have answered THE question. Note that the other three options can be clustered to be findings with not data in the stem to support.

4. Correct answer: b

Forty percent of individuals with bulimia experience a weight problem before the behavior starts. It is when they experience weight loss that they may develop this behavior and diagnosis. They have an intense fear of gaining weight, so they engage in binging and

The approach is to read carefully and slowly. If you have no idea of the correct answer, eliminate options *c* and *d,* since they have the absolute phrases, "intense fear" and "exclusively." Eliminate option *a,* since the age on onset is in a developmental period, adolescence, and is not a specific age. Select option *b.*

purging to maintain their weight or to continue weight loss. It occurs in both sexes, with current reports of a greater frequency in females. Clients with anorexia nervosa have a body image disturbance and an intense fear of foods that cause weight gain. Both may begin in adolescence.

5. **Correct answer: b**

Amenorrhea, hypotension, and lanugo, fine downy hair, are more commonly assessed characteristics of individuals with anorexia than anemia. Anemia is more likely to take a longer period of time to develop than the other findings.

Substance Use Disorders

STUDY OUTCOMES

After completing this chapter, the reader will be able to do
the following:

▼ Define substance dependence and abuse.
▼ Discuss the problem of substance use disorders in the health care
  professions.
▼ Describe precipitating stressors to substance use disorders.
▼ Discuss theories of causality of substance use disorders.
▼ Define the major categories of abused substances related to route
  of administration, expected behavioral responses, and behaviors
  related to overdose and to withdrawal syndromes.
▼ Apply the nursing process to clients experiencing substance use
  disorders.

KEY TERMS

Addiction	Psychological and physiological dependence on a substance.
Dual diagnosis	Coexistence of a major psychiatric disorder and a substance use disorder.
Habituation	Psychological craving for a particular substance.
Intoxication	Reversible substance-specific symptoms due to a recent ingestion of a substance.
Potentiation	Combining drugs results in a greater effect (1 + 1 = 3).
Substance dependence	Pattern of repeated use of a substance, which usually results in tolerance, withdrawal, and compulsive drug-taking behavior.
Tolerance	Need for increased amounts of the substance to achieve the desired effect.
Withdrawal	Physiological and/or substance-specific cognitive symptoms when blood levels decrease in an individual with prolonged heavy use of a substance.

CONTENT REVIEW

I. Substance dependence

A. Tolerance and withdrawal occur often but are not necessary for dependence

B. Clients take substance in larger amounts and over longer periods of time than was intended

C. Clients desire to cut down

D. Clients have unsuccessful efforts to decrease or discontinue use

E. Substance dependence consumes much of the client's time

F. Daily activities revolve around a substance

G. Clients continue using a substance despite the problems it creates

II. Substance abuse

A. Clients experience recurrent, significant, harmful consequences related to the repeated use of substances

B. Clients recurrently use substances in physically hazardous situations, such as driving a car

C. Clients have legal problems related to substance use

D. Use is related to client's failure in any role obligations— work, school, home

III. Epidemiology of substance use disorder (DSM IV, 1994)

A. Ranks among the top three most serious health problems in America

B. Use of inhalants has doubled since 1970; use begins by 9 to 12 years of age; peaks in adolescence; less common after 35 years of age; 70 to 80% are male users.

C. Number of cocaine and crack users rose from 8 to 12 million between 1985 and 1988; DSM IV reports of a 1991 study: 12% of the population used cocaine one or more times in lifetime; 3% in the last year; 1% in the last month; 0.2% of population has abused cocaine at some time in their lives.

D. Alcohol use has risen by 10%; 14% of noninstitutionalized adults, ages 15 to 54, had alcohol dependence at some time in their lives.

E. Men outnumber women 2 to 1

IV. Substance use disorders in health care professionals

A. High incidence of alcohol and prescription drug abuse in nurses and physicians

B. 1.7 million nurses are alcoholics

C. Licensure discipline cases often are related to substance abuse

D. Responsibility lies with all nurses to intervene when a coworker is practicing under-the-influence

E. Signs of abuse in professional colleagues
   1. Absenteeism
   2. Tardiness
   3. Sloppy work
   4. Irritability
   5. Medication errors
   6. Seclusiveness

F. Colleagues often work as enablers of the substance abuse professional

V. Theories of causality

A. Disease model
   1. Can be diagnosed as a disease process
   2. Is the cause of other medical and psychiatric problems
   3. Predictable and progressive in course
   4. Is treatable
   5. Genetic predisposition—limited to alcohol versus other substances in available research
   6. Biochemical deficits in the narcotic receptor ligand system

B. **Psychodynamic theory**
 1. Euphoria is escape from depression
 2. Gratification of oral and genital needs
 3. Way to act out anger
 4. Coping mechanism
 5. Symptom of underlying psychopathology
C. **Adaption model**
 1. Attempt to adapt to severe distress
 2. Escape from life crises
 3. Family model
  a. Attempt to relieve family stress
  b. Avoidance of focusing on family by focusing on consequences of drug abuse
  c. Triangulation of parent to substance to avoid marital problems and intimacy
D. **Behavioral theory**
 1. Drug use develops through leaning and modeling and positive reinforcement of mood alteration
 2. Environmental "triggers" elicit craving for the substance
E. **Multicausal theory**
 1. Combination of
  a. Heredity
  b. Psychological structure
  c. Sociocultural factors
 2. Mediating factors that prevent disorder
  a. Social class
  b. Family dynamics
  c. Support systems

VI. Precipitating stressors (Figure 11-1)
A. **Adolescence**
 1. Rebellion
 2. Peer group pressure
B. **Pleasure seeking**
 1. Creates pleasure state
 2. Decreases physical and emotional pain
C. **Sociocultural stressors**
 1. Tension reduction
 2. Socially approved
D. **Group influence and peer pressure**
E. **Depression**
F. **Loss/grieving**

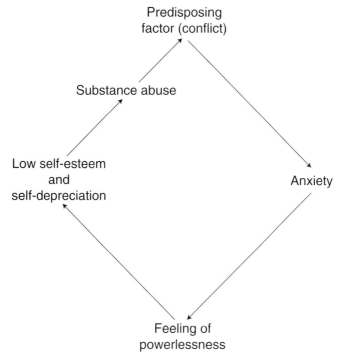

Figure 11-1. The cycle of substance abuse. (From Stuart G and Sundeen S: *Principles and practice of psychiatric nursing,* ed 4, St Louis, 1991, Mosby.)

VII. Seven dysfunctional behaviors associated with substance abuse

  A. **Manipulation**
     1. Getting needs met at expense of others
     2. Insensitivity to self and others

  B. **Impulsiveness**
     1. Act suddenly without thought
     2. Decreases anxiety

  C. **Anger**
     1. Anesthetizes feelings
     2. Physical and verbal abuse
     3. Act out feelings

  D. **Avoidance**
     1. Physical and emotional distancing
     2. Avoidance of relationships
     3. Lack of social skills
     4. Fear of self-disclosure
     5. Avoidance of feelings

    E. Grandiosity: sense of self-importance—require special privileges or treatment

    F. Denial
1. Main dynamic in substance dependence
2. Others enable this dynamic to continue
3. Blame everything but the substance

    G. Codependence
1. Extreme emotional, social, or physical focus on another person
2. Individuals modify their behaviors in response to others
3. Often clients and family members are codependent
4. Attempts to control others, such as through drinking behavior
5. Low self-esteem
6. Compulsive behavior
7. No thoughts, feelings, ideas of own
8. Feels depressed
9. Feels grandiose
10. Hypervigilant for sign of problems with the substance (Modified from Haber et al, 1992)

VIII. Alcohol

    A. Alcohol dependence
1. Drinking behavior interferes with activities of daily living
2. Drinking adversely affects interpersonal relationships
3. Episodic excessive drinking or addiction
4. Physical dependence—biological need for alcohol to avoid physical withdrawal symptoms
5. Psychological dependence—craving for the subjective effect of alcohol

    B. Alcohol is a central nervous system depressant

    C. Once alcohol is absorbed into blood stream, it affects all body tissues

    D. Immediate effect is on brain

    E. Relationship exists between blood alcohol levels and behavior in a nontolerant drinker

    F. Alcohol equivalencies
1. Wine—4 ounces equal 12% alcohol
2. Beer—12 ounces equal 12% alcohol
3. Hard liquor—1 ounce equals 48% alcohol

    G. Warning signs of a problem with alcohol
1. Sneaking drinks

    2. Morning drinking

    3. Blackouts

    4. Binge drinking

    5. Arguments about drinking

    6. Missing time at work

    7. Increased tolerance to alcohol

    8. Intoxication—blood alcohol level greater than or equal to 0.1% (Modified from Stuart and Sundeen, 1991)

H. Physical symptoms of alcohol dependence

    1. Fatty liver

    2. Hepatitis

    3. Cirrhosis of liver

    4. Esophagitis

    5. Gastritis

    6. Pancreatitis

    7. Cardiomyopathy

    8. Anemias

    9. Immune system dysfunctions

    10. Peripheral neuropathy

    11. Brain damage

    12. Telangiectasia—dilation of a group of small blood vessels, usually on face

    13. Acne rosacea—skin disease of nose, face, chin

    14. Elevated SGOT

    15. Low hematocrit

    16. Low potassium and phosphorous

    17. Wide swings in blood sugar

I. Psychological symptoms of alcohol dependence

    1. Depression

    2. Hostility

    3. Suspiciousness

    4. Denial of problem

    5. Rationalization

    6. Irritability

    7. Isolation

    8. Decrease in inhibitions

    9. Decrease in self-esteem

J. Symptoms of alcohol withdrawal

    1. Begin 6 to 8 hours after drinking has ended or decreased below the normal consumption

    2. Last 5 to 7 days and has four stages

3. Stage 1—6 to 8 hours after last ingestion or significant decrease in usual consumption of alcohol (symptoms in order of appearance)
   a. Anxiety
   b. Anorexia
   c. Insomnia
   d. Tremors—hand, eye, tongue
   e. Hyperalertness
   f. "Internal shaking"
   g. Nausea
   h. Vomiting
   i. Depression
   j. Headache
   k. Insomnia
   l. Weakness
   m. Increased blood pressure
   n. Tachycardia—heart rates range from 120 to 140
   o. Diaphoresis
4. Stage 2—8 to 12 hours after the last ingestion or significant decrease in usual consumption of alcohol (symptoms in order of appearance)
   a. Profound confusion
   b. Gross tremors
   c. Nervousness
   d. Hyperactivity
   e. Disorientation
   f. Illusions
   g. Nightmares
   h. Auditory and visual hallucinations
5. Stage 3—12 to 48 hours after the last ingestion or significant decrease in usual consumption of alcohol
   a. All of symptoms of stages 1 and 2
   b. Severe hallucinations
   c. Grand mal seizures ("rum" fits)
6. Stage 4—3 to 5 days after the last ingestion or significant decrease in usual consumption of alcohol
   a. Delirium tremors (DTs)
   b. Confusion
   c. Severe psychomotor activity
   d. Agitation
   e. Sleeplessness
   f. Hallucinations

      g. Uncontrolled tachycardia

      h. Medical emergency—client may die despite treatment in this stage

  7. Treatment of alcohol withdrawal

      a. Seizure and hallucination prevention: magnesium sulfate 50% solution and PO Librium or Ativan

      b. Treatment for malnutrition: thiamine 50 to 100 mg IM

      c. Seizure precautions

      d. Hydration

K. Problems associated with chronic alcohol dependence

  1. Vitamin deficiencies: Vitamin B—peripheral neuropathies

  2. Thiamine deficiency

      a. Alcohol-induced, persistent amnestic disorder, also called Korsakoff's syndrome—severe memory problems

      b. Wernicke's encephalopathy—findings

         (1) Confusion

         (2) Ataxia

         (3) Abnormal eye movements

IX. Behaviors associated with abuse of other substances

A. Psychotomimetics

  1. Abused by adolescents and young adults

  2. Induce state like psychosis

  3. LSD (lysergic acid diethylamide)

  4. PCP (phencyclidine)

  5. THC (tetrahydrocarnabinal)

      a. Active ingredient of marijuana

      b. Mescaline

      c. Psilocybin

      d. Peyote

  6. Effects

      a. Distorted perceptions

      b. Heightened sense of awareness

      c. Grandiosity

      d. Hallucinations

      e. Mystical experiences

      f. Distortions of time and space

  7. No physical or psychological dependence

  8. No withdrawal syndrome when discontinued

  9. Nursing considerations

      a. "Bad trip" may result in panic, unpredictable behavior, psychotic behaviors

   b. "Flashbacks" may occur for several months after use stops

   c. May harm self when under influence

 B. **Opiates**

   1. Types of drugs

    a. Opium

    b. Heroin

    c. Meperidine

    d. Morphine

    e. Codeine

    f. Methadone—used for treatment of addictions

   2. Behaviors

    a. Mental and physical deterioration

    b. Illegal behaviors to obtain drugs or money for drugs

    c. High risk for infection if taken intravenously

     (1) HIV (human immunodeficiency virus): virus that causes AIDS (acquired immunodeficiency syndrome)

     (2) Shared needles

     (3) Blood transferred from one person to another

     (4) Babies delivered infected with HIV

   3. Effects

    a. Decreased response to pain

    b. Respiratory depression

    c. Constriction of pupils

    d. Slowing of digestive processes

    e. Euphoria

    f. Apathy

    g. Detachment from others

    h. Impaired judgment

   4. Withdrawal

    a. Uncomfortable

    b. Usually not life threatening

    c. Use Methadone to help with withdrawal

    d. Anxiety

    e. Yawning

    f. Diaphoresis

    g. Cramps

    h. Rhinorrhea

    i. Achiness

    j. Muscular twitching

    k. Anorexia

    l. Insomnia

   m. Hypertension
   n. Increased temperature
   o. Increased respirations
   p. Restlessness
   q. Nausea and vomiting
   r. Diarrhea
  5. Overdosage
   a. Coma
   b. Respiratory depression
   c. Death

C. Barbiturates
  1. Types
   a. Barbital
   b. Amobarbital (Amytal)
   c. Phenobarbital
   d. Pentobarbital (Nembutal)
   e. Secobarbital (Seconal)
   f. Butabarbital
  2. Action
   a. Depressant
   b. Sedative
   c. Hypnotic
  3. Physical and psychological dependence
  4. Effects
   a. Euphoria
   b. Depression
   c. Hostility
   d. Decreased inhibitions
   e. Impaired judgment
   f. Lack of coordination
   g. Slurring of speech
  5. Tolerance develops
  6. Withdrawal
   a. May be dangerous
   b. Postural hypotension
   c. Tachycardia
   d. Increased temperature
   e. Insomnia
   f. Tremors
   g. Agitation
   h. Apprehension
   i. Weakness

        j. Grand mal seizures

        k. Psychosis

D. **Amphetamines**

  1. Stimulants

  2. Alertness

  3. Extra energy

  4. Types

      a. Caffeine

      b. Amphetamines

      c. Cocaine

      d. Methamphetamine

      e. Benzphetamine

  5. Uses

      a. Obesity

      b. Narcolepsy

      c. Hyperactive children (paradoxical calming effect)

  6. Effects

      a. Euphoria

      b. Hyperactivity

      c. Insomnia

      d. Anorexia

      e. Weight loss

      f. Tachycardia

      g. Hypertension

      h. Psychotic behavior

  7. Psychological dependence

  8. No physical dependence

  9. Tolerance

  10. Withdrawal

      a. "Crash"

      b. Depression

      c. Lack of energy

E. **Cocaine**

  1. Symbol of sophistication

  2. Stimulant

  3. Freebasing—smoking drug after it has been chemically processed

  4. Crack—result of above processing

  5. Short-acting

      a. 60 to 90 minutes (inhaled)

      b. 30 to 60 minutes (injected)

      c. 5 minutes (smoked—crack form)

    6. Effects
       a. Euphoria
       b. Energetic
       c. Self-confident
       d. Sociable
    7. Action
       a. Blocks reuptake of norepinephrine and dopamine—results in euphoria
       b. Results in vasoconstriction of various body organs
    8. Sudden death has been associated with cocaine abuse

F. **Marijuana—general effects**
    1. Altered state of awareness
    2. Relaxation
    3. Mild euphoria
    4. Decreased inhibition
    5. Decreased motivation from prolonged use
    6. Possible psychosis
    7. Physiological effects
       a. Slowed reflexes
       b. Drying of mucous membranes
       c. Reddening of eyes
       d. Pulmonary changes similar to those from tobacco
       e. Increased likelihood of pregnancy
       f. Developmental problems in fetus

G. **Antianxiety drugs**
    1. Types
       a. Librium
       b. Valium
       c. Xanax
       d. Antivan
    2. Physically and psychologically addictive
    3. Tolerance does occur
    4. Effects
       a. Relaxation
       b. Confidence
       c. Drowsiness
       d. Hypotension
       e. Ataxia
    5. Withdrawal
       a. Seizures
       b. Similar to that from benzodiazepines

X. Nursing process with clients experiencing substance use disorder

A. Assessment
1. Cage screening test
   a. C—Have you ever felt the need to CUT down on your drug use?
   b. A—Have you ever been ANNOYED at criticism of your drug use?
   c. G—Have you ever felt GUILTY about something you have done when you have been high from drugs?
   d. E—Have you ever had an EYE opener (taken drugs) first thing in the morning to get going (avoid withdrawal symptoms)?
2. Physical
   a. Patterns of use
      (1) Quantity
      (2) Frequency
      (3) Circumstances: may use same format to ask about drug use
      (4) When was the last time you had any alcoholic beverages?
      (5) What beverages do you drink?
      (6) How many drinks do you have?
      (7) Where and with whom do you drink?
   b. Physical symptoms
      (1) Withdrawal symptoms pertinent to substance used
      (2) Laboratory tests (BAL—blood alcohol level)
      (3) Liver function
3. Psychological
   a. Denial
   b. Rationalization
   c. Paranoid ideas
   d. Confusion
   e. Sedation
   f. Belligerence
   g. Grandiosity
   h. Unpredictable behavior
B. Nursing diagnoses
1. Ineffective individual coping
2. Ineffective denial
3. Powerlessness related to substance
4. Self-esteem disturbance

    5. Sleep pattern disturbance
    6. Impaired social interaction
    7. Altered thought process
       a. Paranoia
       b. Confusion
       c. Memory impairment
       d. Delusions
    8. Sensory/perceptual alteration
       a. Hallucinations
       b. Illusions
    9. Anxiety
  10. Risk for violence
  11. Dysfunctional family process
  12. Hopelessness
  13. Grief
  14. Alteration in comfort
  15. Alteration in nutritional status

C. Nursing interventions
    1. Manipulation
       a. Hold client firmly to reasonable limits
       b. Consistently enforce rules with reasonable consequences for breaking rules
    2. Impulsiveness
       a. Hold client accountable for behaviors
       b. Encourage feedback from other clients, family, etc. related to client's behaviors
       c. Enforce consequences for behaviors
    3. Anger
       a. Set limits on verbal and physical abuse
       b. Encourage timeout if losing control
       c. Encourage client to identify and discuss feelings
       d. Identify with client situations that precipitate angry feelings
    4. Avoidance
       a. Encourage client to participate in unit activities such as games
       b. Encourage self-exploration and ownership of feelings
    5. Grandiosity
       a. Help client identify similarities between self and others
       b. Explore realistic strengths and weaknesses
       c. Explore ways to realistically have client's needs met without sense of entitlement
    6. Withdrawal—interventions based on substance and symptoms

7. Overdose
   a. Identify drug
   b. Narcotics—give nalorphine (Narcan), a narcotic antagonist; usually IV push; repeat if needed. Caution—observe for signs of withdrawal.
   c. Benzodiazepines—give flumazenit (Mazicon), IV push, repeat to a maximum of 3 mg
8. Toxic psychosis
   a. Users of LSD and PCP
   b. Looks like schizophrenia
   c. Provide safe environment
   d. Allow minimal stimuli
   e. Calm, empathetic, reassurring behaviors
   f. Reorientation
   g. Provide for safety—adequate staff
   h. Give cranberry juice—acidifies urine and increases excretion of PCP
   i. Implement gastric lavage if necessary
9. Antabuse therapy
   a. Used for alcoholic dependence
   b. Drug sensitizes client to alcohol so a negative physiological response occurs if alcohol is ingested
      (1) Headache
      (2) Nausea
      (3) Vomiting
      (4) Flushing
      (5) Hypotension
      (6) Tachycardia
      (7) Dyspnea
      (8) Diaphoresis
      (9) Chest pain
      (10) Palpitations
      (11) Dizziness
      (12) Confusion
      (13) Respiratory collapse
      (14) Cardiac collapse
      (15) Unconsciousness
      (16) Convulsions
      (17) Death
   c. Client must be educated as to effects and agree to abstain from alcohol
   d. Alcohol-containing substances must also be avoided
      (1) Cough medicines

       (2) Rubbing compounds
       (3) Vinegars
       (4) Aftershave lotions
       (5) Mouthwashes
    e. Must avoid drinking for 14 days after antabuse therapy has been discontinued; if no avoidance for 14 days, client has risk to exhibit negative physiological responses

10. Recidivism
    a. Usually chronic with periods of exacerbation and partial or full remission
    b. Alcohol
       (1) 20% achieve long-term sobriety even without treatment
       (2) 65% remain abstinent first year after treatment
    c. Amphetamines
       (1) Chronic use becomes unpleasant for clients
       (2) Usually clients decrease or stop use after 8 to 10 years
    d. Cannabis—pattern of chronic use
    e. Opioids—relapse following abstinence is common
    f. Self-help groups effective in preventing relapse
    g. Frustrating for nurse dealing with clients experiencing substance use
       (1) Avoid rejection of a returning client; it is not helpful
       (2) Focus on beginning again
       (3) Assess what did not work
       (4) Plan new strategies

11. Family counseling
    a. Focus on codependent and enabling behaviors
    b. Encourage direct expression of feelings
    c. Explore boundary issues

12. Refer to self-help groups, 12-step programs

13. Community treatment programs
    a. Individual counseling
    b. Group counseling
    c. Family counseling
    d. Vocational counseling
    e. Drug and health education
    f. Methadone maintenance—opiate addicts
    g. Peer group pressure

14. Refer client to transitional living programs
    a. Halfway houses
    b. Transition between detoxification and independence
    c. 12-step programs
    d. Vocational rehabilitation

    D. Treatment outcomes
1. Commitment to abstinence
2. Ongoing treatment
   a. Peer support
   b. Improved coping skills
   c. Healthier family relationships
   d. Continued 12-step programs
   e. Psychotherapy—exploration of underlying personality structure

    E. Prevention of substance use
1. Improved social conditions
2. Education—schools, legislative action
3. Increased interpersonal and social skills
4. Increased self-esteem

REVIEW QUESTIONS

1. A young, pregnant client has a history of addiction to heroin. What other finding should be investigated for?
   a. Positive for HIV
   b. Syphilis
   c. Tuberculosis
   d. Bacteremia

2. The client with alcohol withdrawal delirium has disorientation and threatening hallucinations. At this time what other clinical finding would the nurse find in this client?
   a. Increased alertness
   b. Seizure activity
   c. Agitation
   d. Cerebellar ataxia

3. The drying out period during which the client is withdrawing from alcohol is called
   a. Antibuse therapy
   b. Detoxification
   c. Medication therapy
   d. Withdrawal syndrome

4. The most common defense mechanism used by the alcoholic client is
   a. Sublimation
   b. Compensation
   c. Denial
   d. Rationalization

5. A client is experiencing alcohol withdrawal delirium. The nurse should implement which priority action?
   a. Discuss the benefits of Alcoholics Anonymous meetings
   b. Keep the client awake and oriented
   c. Monitor blood pressure and pulse
   d. Record hourly output

ANSWERS, RATIONALES, AND TEST-TAKING TIPS

Rationales	Test-Taking Tips

1. **Correct answer: a**

The heroin addict is most likely to have had shared needles with a high risk of acquiring HIV. There is not enough information in the stem to select the other options.

Use your knowledge that IV users have the higher risk of acquiring HIV.

2. **Correct answer: c**

Options *a* and *d* are not findings in alcohol withdrawal delirium. Seizure activity may occur but not until the more severe stages. There is no information in the stem to indicate that the client is in the severe phase.

The most important approach to selection of the correct answer is to read the question and the responses carefully to note the time frame. When the client is disoriented with threatening hallucinations agitation is most likely rather than seizures.

3. **Correct answer: b**

Detoxification is the "drying out" period. This is the removal of alcohol from the client, with the prevention of withdrawal findings by the use of alternative substances and a gradual withdrawal. Antibuse therapy is used after detoxification to prevent clients from returning to alcohol. Medication therapy is too general of a response to be the correct answer; it may be one approach in the detoxification process. Withdrawal syndrome is what happens when the client stops ingesting alcohol.

The key words in the stem are "the drying out period. Of the given responses, option *b* makes most sense.

4. **Correct answer: c**

Denial is a primitive defense mechanism. It is lack of awareness of external happenings and is used primarily by alcoholics to deny that they have a drinking problem. Sublimation is acceptance of a socially approved substitute goal for a drive whose normal channel of expression is blocked. Compensation is the process by which a person makes up for a deficiency in image of self by strongly emphasizing some other feature that the person regards as an asset. Rationalization is the offering of a socially acceptable or apparently logical explanation to justify or make acceptable otherwise unacceptable impulses, feelings, behaviors, and motives.

If you have no idea of the correct answer, *go with what you know;* the most common defense mechanism you most likely know is denial; select it.

5. **Correct answer: c**

Alcoholic withdrawal tremens, previously called delirium tremens, is a life-threatening event. The client may experience acute psychosis, as well as elevated blood pressure and pulse rate. It is a priority to monitor vital signs and level of consciousness to prevent any further complications. However, the client is not purposefully stimulated to be kept awake.

If you have no idea of the correct answer, eliminate option *a,* since a client in delirium will be incapable of discussing anything. Read option *b* carefully to note how it is phrased; it would cause the client to be more agitated. Note that this statement does not mean to monitor the client's level of consciousness. The best choice between options *c* and *d* is *c,* since cardiac function is a priority over renal function in this client.

Urine output is monitored but not every hour, which would require an indwelling urinary catheter and drainage system and cause the client to be more agitated.

Abusive/Self-Destructive Behavior

STUDY OUTCOMES

After completing this chapter, the reader will be able to do the following:

▼ Identify types of abuse and neglect.
▼ Describe characteristics of individuals at risk for becoming victims or perpetrators of abuse.
▼ Discuss theories on the etiology of family violence.
▼ Describe common reactions of survivors of rape or sexual assault.
▼ Describe responses of survivors of family violence.
▼ Define physical and psychological abuse, neglect, and exploitation.
▼ Apply the nursing process in working with both victims and victimizers.

KEY TERMS

Exploitation	Use of the victim for selfish purposes and/or financial profit (Haber et al, 1992).
Family violence	Includes physical and emotional abuse of children, child neglect, spouse battering, marital rape, and elder abuse (Stuart and Sundeen, 1995).
Physical abuse	Deliberate violent actions that inflict pain and/or nonaccidental injury, which may cause permanent or temporary disfigurement or death (Haber et al, 1992).
Physical neglect	Deliberate deprivation or nonprovision of necessary and societal-available resources (Haber et al, 1992).
Psychological abuse	Deliberate and willful destruction or significant impairment of a person's sense of competence through behaviors that have a negative impact on the victim's self esteem, psychosocial development, and social relationships (Haber et al, 1992).
Psychological neglect	Psychosocial unavailability and caretaking that lacks warmth and sensitive, personalized attention (Haber et al, 1992).
Sexual abuse	Use of victim for sexual gratification when the victim is either unable or unwilling to consent.

CONTENT REVIEW

I. Theories related to abuse, neglect, exploitation

A. Instinct theory—innate aggressive tendencies

B. Genetic theory—Y chromosome connection to aggressive impulses

C. Neurophysiologic theory—increased levels of neurotransmitters (norepinephrine, dopamine, and serotonin) connected with aggression

D. Brain lesion theory
   1. Tumors
   2. Seizures

E. Psychosis
   1. Delusions
   2. Hallucinations

F. Intrapsychic theory
   1. Victims identify with victimizers in order to survive
   2. Victims internalize victimizers and become themselves aggressive

G. **Intrapersonal theory**
1. Impaired ability to relate to others
2. Impaired superego development
3. Self-centered
4. Impulsive
5. Devalue others
6. Susceptible to rage

H. **Family systems theory**
1. Multigenerational transmission
2. Triangles
3. Level of differentiation

I. **Social learning theory**
1. Learned ways of coping with stress and frustration
2. Passive response to abuse

J. **Media influence—glorification of violence in newspapers, advertisements, toys, games, and television**

K. **Alcohol abuse—decreases control over impulsive behavior**

L. **Cocaine abuse**
1. Paranoid thinking
2. Compulsive need for drug

M. **Hallucinogen abuse**
1. Disorientation
2. Misinterpretation of reality

II. Violence and aggression

A. **Violence**
1. Physical force
2. Unjust strength. Example: husband who is physically stronger beats up his much smaller wife.
3. Power
4. Consequences for perpetrators and victims
5. Arouses fear in others
6. Threat to personal safety
7. Trauma remains vivid in dreams and thoughts
8. May be premeditated or spontaneous
9. Intense hatred and rage

B. **Aggression**
1. Natural drive—Freud believed aggression to be an id impulse
2. Motivating force—impulses and feelings are converted into action
3. If not controlled or sublimated
   a. Harmful
   b. Destructive

4. Can be constructive or destructive
5. Expression is learned reaction
6. Violence—destructive aggressive drive

III. Anger

A. Feeling of annoyance or displeasure
B. Natural feeling
C. The development of anger (Figure 12-1)
D. May be displaced onto object or person
E. Used to avoid anxiety
F. Anger gives feeling of power in situations in which person feels out of control
G. Result of frustration
H. Characteristic findings of anger
   1. Muscle rigidity
   2. Flushed face
   3. Pacing
   4. Pounding
   5. Stomping
   6. Loud voice
   7. Speeded up body movements
   8. Glaring
I. Assessment findings for violence potential in response to anger
   1. History of violence
   2. Poor impulse control
   3. History of self-harm
   4. Temper tantrums
   5. Low tolerance of frustration
   6. Increased pacing
   7. Increased agitation
   8. Verbal threats of violence
   9. Defiance
   10. Argumentation
J. Nursing interventions for the angry client
   1. Set limits on behavior
   2. Provide safe outlets for expressing anger
   3. Provide safety for clients and others
   4. Acknowledge anger
   5. Model expression of anger
   6. Listen actively
   7. Help deal with consequences of anger

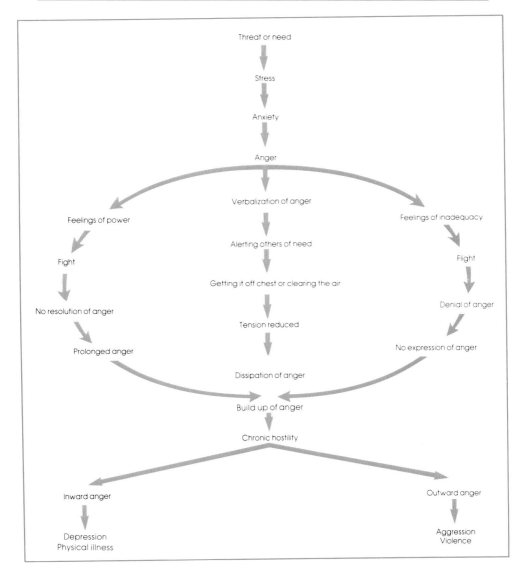

Figure 12-1. The development and expression of anger. (From Rawlins R, Williams S and Beck: *Mental health-Psychiatric nursing: A holistic life-cycle approach*, ed 3, St Louis, 1993, Mosby.)

    8. Teach assertiveness
    9. Provide positive feedback when client is appropriately expressing anger
  10. Help resolve conflicts and solve problems
  11. Apply physical restraints if necessary. Restraint guidelines
      a. Physical and verbal threats from client
      b. Hypersensitivity of client to environmental stimuli

      c. Physical assault to self, others, or environment
      d. Help client gain physical control
      e. Physician orders required
      f. RN supervision required
      g. Adequate number of staff required

   12. Seclusion
      a. Client behaviors that require seclusion (highest priority to lowest priority)
         (1) Need for protection of self or others
         (2) Destructiveness to physical environment
         (3) Increasing agitation
         (4) Hyperactivity
      b. Care provider actions (in order of sequence)
         (1) Use short, simple, direct statements
         (2) May give medication to calm client
         (3) Remove dangerous articles
         (4) Have room prepared in advance
         (5) Use seclusion as a last resort

IV. Family violence

  A. Demographics
     1. All socioeconomic levels
     2. All educational, racial, occupational, gender, and religious groups
  B. Victimizers—characteristics
     1. Impaired self-esteem
     2. Strong, unrealistic dependency needs
     3. Immaturity
     4. Self-absorption
     5. Narcissistic
     6. Suspicious
     7. History of sexual abuse during childhood
     8. Perceive victims as property
     9. Believe they are entitled to abuse victim
  C. Victims—characteristics
     1. Feels like a captive in the system
     2. Dependent
     3. Helpless
     4. Powerless
     5. Blame themselves
     6. Low self-esteem
     7. Depressed

D. Family system (Clinical Example 12-1). Assess for an indication of family dysfunction

1. Low level of differentiation (see section on family systems theory in Chapter 6, pp. 91-93)
2. Unable to meet own or others' needs
3. Characteristics
   a. Impermeable boundaries to outsiders
   b. No one is aware what is happening in the family
   c. When outsiders try to enter, family feels assaulted. Example: abusive father convinces daughter to keep the violence a secret.
   d. Socially isolated family members
   e. Pain and desperation among family members
   f. Family members expect other family members to meet their needs, but no one capable of doing this
   g. Parents usually married young
   h. Lack of autonomy among family members
   i. Lack of trust among family members
   j. Absence of (in the family)
      (1) Humor
      (2) Flexibility
      (3) Caring
      (4) Empathy
      (5) Excitement
      (6) Productivity
      (7) Clear communication
      (8) Intimacy
4. Family violence
   a. May be an attempt for closeness and companionship

Clinical Example 12-1. Family System Dysfunction

Arnold has been passed over for promotions on numerous occasions and has made no friends at work during 10 years of employment at the same company. His wife returned to work to help family finances. She was promoted rapidly, and her managerial position required frequent travel abroad. Arnold's self-concept decreased with his wife's successes, and he turned to his 5-year-old daughter for companionship, sexual gratification, and enhancement of his self-esteem.

Modified from Haber et al: *Comprehensive psychiatric nursing,* ed 4, St Louis, 1992, Mosby.

  b. May provide release of frustration

  c. Allows for coping with a problematic world

 5. Conflict

  a. Expressed through violence, aggression

  b. Power struggles

  c. Confusion of caring with violence

  d. Sexuality and aggression become fused—rape

  e. Cycle of response to decrease stress

 6. Focus on present

  a. Minimal awareness of past or future

  b. Long-range goal-directed behaviors not evident

 7. Financial problems

 8. Early marriages

 9. Lack of parenting skills

10. Lack of underlying normal growth and development

11. Communication characteristics within family

  a. Mixed messages

  b. Lack of direct communication

  c. Decreased communication outside of family—family secrets

12. Values and beliefs

  a. Violence is normal

  b. Victim is responsible for abuse

  c. Problems are solved through violence

13. Abuse of power

  a. Abuser tells others they are worthless

  b. Threats of abandonment

  c. Stereotyping of behaviors

   (1) Woman's work is in home

   (2) Children are not to be heard

   (3) Older siblings may punish younger ones

   (4) Elders have little to contribute

14. The cycle of violence (Figure 12-2) (in order of occurrence)

  a. Tension-building phase

   (1) Minor assaults

   (2) Verbal assaults

   (3) Threats

   (4) Victim attempts to comply

   (5) Alienation from support systems

  b. Explosion

   (1) Major trauma

   (2) Destructiveness

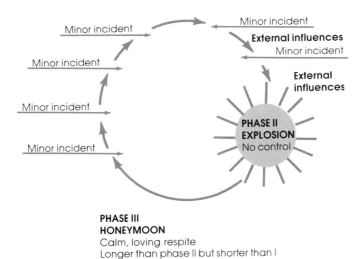

PHASE I
TENSION BUILDING
Limited control

Minor incident

Minor incident

Minor incident

Minor incident

Minor incident

Minor incident
External influences
Minor incident

External influences

PHASE II
EXPLOSION
No control

PHASE III
HONEYMOON
Calm, loving respite
Longer than phase II but shorter than I

Figure 12-2. Walker's cycle theory of battering. (From Rawlins R, Williams S and Beck: *Mental health-Psychiatric nursing: A holistic life-cycle approach,* ed 3, St Louis, 1993, Mosby.)

        (3) Lack of control
        (4) Victims protect themselves
        (5) Victims underplay the severity
   c. Honeymoon period
        (1) Tenderness
        (2) Love
        (3) Truce
 E. Types of family violence
     1. Child abuse or neglect
       a. Physical or mental injury
       b. Sexual abuse
       c. Negligence
       d. Maltreatment
       e. Under 18 years of age
       f. Usually is the person responsible for child's welfare
       g. Mandatory reporting is required by nurses for confirmed or suspected cases
       h. Vulnerable population because of victim's dependence on care provider
       i. Cyclical, repetitive acts of abuse arc typical

  j. Assessment findings
    (1) Client reported
      (a) Night terrors
      (b) Chronic fatigue
      (c) Somniloquy (talking during sleep)
      (d) Enuresis (incontinence of urine)
      (e) Insomnia
      (f) Increased sleeping
      (g) Weight loss or gain
    (2) Observations by care providers
      (a) External signs of trauma
      (b) Scarring
      (c) Head injuries
      (d) Immunizations and dental care lacking
      (e) Fear in the presence of parent(s) or careprovider
    (3) Exams/procedures to collect data
      (a) Ear exams
      (b) Ophthalmoscopic examinations
      (c) Gynecological exams
      (d) Tests for sexually transmitted diseases
      (e) X-rays
      (f) Tests for urinary tract infections
  k. Nursing diagnoses
    (1) Ineffective family coping
    (2) Anxiety related to parents' abusive behaviors
    (3) Fear
    (4) Self-esteem disturbance
    (5) Sleep pattern disturbances
  l. Interventions
    (1) Protect child from further harm
    (2) Move slowly around child
    (3) Use lights; avoid loud noises
    (4) Keep child near center of activity
    (5) Keep at eye level of child for communication
    (6) Have child participate in decisions about care
    (7) Educate family on alternate ways to express feelings of hostility and frustration
    (8) Refer parents to parenting classes
    (9) Do not rescue child from parents
    (10) Reassure child that he/she is loved and not responsible for parents' behaviors

(11) Encourage family to connect with community support systems such as Parents Anonymous

(12) Give parents numbers of crisis hotlines

(13) Reassure child that he/she is not a bad person

(14) Collaborate with physician and authorities to report suspected or confirmed child abuse cases

2. Elder abuse
   a. Family history of dysfunction
      (1) Alcohol abuse
      (2) Unemployment
      (3) Change in living arrangement, such as when a son and family move into mother's home
      (4) Burden of caring for ill older parent
      (5) Isolation
      (6) Rigid, compulsive, inflexible
      (7) History of abusive relationships
   b. Types of abuse
      (1) Physical—infliction of pain or injury
      (2) Sexual
      (3) Psychological—infliction of mental anguish by demeaning, name calling, insulting
      (4) Financial/material—exploitation using assets, funds for personal gain
   c. Types of neglect
      (1) Passive—unintentional failure to caretaking of elder person's physical, emotional or financial needs.
      (2) Active—abandonment, denial of food, shelter, clothing, medical assistance, personal needs, isolation; an intentional neglect
   d. Assessment findings
      (1) Physical abuse
          (a) Fractures
          (b) Welts
          (c) Lacerations
          (d) Punctures
          (e) Burns
          (f) Bruises
              (i) Shape similar to an object (belt marks, fingers)
              (ii) Bilateral on upper arms
              (iii) Clustered on trunk

    (2) Sexual abuse
        (a) Torn, stained, or bloody underclothing
        (b) Difficulty in walking or sitting
        (c) Pain, itching, bruising, or bleeding in genital area
        (d) Unexplained venereal disease or genital infections
    (3) Psychological abuse
        (a) Confusion
        (b) Excessive fears
        (c) Sleep disorders
        (d) Change in appetite
        (e) Unusual weight gain or loss
        (f) Loss of interest in self, activities, or environment
        (g) Ambivalence
        (h) Withdrawal
        () Agitation
    (4) Financial abuse
        (a) Inaccurate, confused, or no knowledge of finances
        (b) Unexplained inability to pay bills
        (c) Disparity between income/assets and lifestyle
        (d) Fear when discussing finances
    (5) Neglect
        (a) Dehydration
        (b) Malnutrition
        (c) Hypo/hyperthermia
        (d) Excessive dirt or odor
        (e) Inadequate or inappropriate clothing
        (f) Absence of eyeglasses, hearing aids, dentures
        (g) Signs of excess drugging
        (h) Decubitus ulcers
  e. Common themes and issues in elder abuse
    (1) Suspected victims may attempt to dismiss physical injuries as accidental
    (2) Abusers may prevent victims from receiving proper medical care to avoid discovery
    (3) Victims may be care providers for the abusers
    (4) Abusers and victims may have unrealistic expectations of each other
    (5) Abusers may resist allowing outsiders to provide services in home
    (6) Victims and abusers often live in same household

   (7) Abusers may be dependent on victim for living expenses

   (8) Victims are often socially isolated

   (9) Mistreatment often increases in severity and frequency over time

   (10) Several types of mistreatment may occur simultaneously

   (11) Denial of mistreatment by victims and abusers is common

 f. Interventions with the victim

   (1) Document observations and indicators of mistreatment

   (2) Provide information related to emergency community resources

   (3) Explore alternative living arrangements—begin with least restrictive and disruptive change

    (a) Arrange for trusted significant other to stay with patient

    (b) Utilize police to remove abuser and obtain order of protection

    (c) Arrange temporary or permanent alternative residence

    (d) Arrange nursing home placement if appropriate

   (4) Assist with financial management protection

    (a) Direct bank deposit

    (b) Joint bank account

    (c) Power of attorney

   (5) Encourage mistreatment counseling

    (a) Issues to explore

     (i) Self-blame

     (ii) Isolation

     (iii) Low self-esteem

    (b) Support groups

    (c) Couple or family counseling

   (6) Assist with legal procedures

    (a) Order of protection

    (b) Police reports

    (c) Court-ordered counseling

   (7) Refer to Protective Services for Adults (PSA)

 g. Nursing interventions with the abuser

   (1) Arrange counseling and treatment

    (a) Individual or group

        (b) Couple or family counseling

        (c) Support groups

        (d) Drug and alcohol treatment programs

        (e) Vocational counseling and job placement

        (f) Coping skills educational groups

    (2) Arrange respite care

        (a) Adult day care or home respite

        (b) Help in home

            (i) Housekeeper

            (ii) Meals-on-wheels

    (3) Provide education

        (a) Short-term and long-term effects of mistreatment

        (b) Alternatives to violence

    (4) Facilitate a change in living arrangements

        (a) Other living arrangements for abuser

        (b) Limit or cease contact with elder

(Modified from Mount Sinai/Victim Services Agency Elder Abuse Project, 1988)

3. Spouse abuse

    a. Often age 18 or older

    b. Involves a relationship with a spouse or a partner

    c. Commonly an intentional act of physical violence

    d. No uniform laws mandating reporting

    e. Often happens first during a pregnancy

    f. Abused spouse/partner reluctant to reveal cause of injuries

    g. Abused spouse/partner often blamed for not leaving

    h. Assessment findings of abused spouse/partner

        (1) Eating disorders

        (2) Insomnia

        (3) Fatigue

        (4) Headaches

        (5) Hypertension

        (6) Palpitations

        (7) Hyperventilation

        (8) Depression

        (9) Suicidal thoughts

        (10) Flat or inappropriate affect

        (11) Guilt

        (12) Fear

        (13) Social isolation

    i. Common injuries from abuse
- (1) Facial injuries
- (2) Head injuries
- (3) Fractures of upper extremities
- (4) Joint tenderness
- (5) Strangulation marks on neck
- (6) Cigarette burns
- (7) Spontaneous abortion
- (8) Human bite marks
- (9) Trauma to genitalia

    j. Nursing diagnoses for abused individual
- (1) Anxiety
- (2) Pain
- (3) Ineffective coping
- (4) Disturbance in self-concept
- (5) Social isolation
- (6) Sleep pattern disturbance
- (7) Alteration in nutritional status

    k. Nursing interventions for abused spouse/partner
- (1) Offer protection
- (2) Relieve of childcare responsibilities
- (3) Facilitate the expression of feelings
  - (a) Ambivalence
  - (b) Guilt
  - (c) Anger
- (4) Help victim make own decisions regarding whether to stay or leave
- (5) Support decisions of client
- (6) Refer client to support groups
- (7) Increase client's self-esteem
- (8) Refer to vocational rehabilitation

V. Rape

- A. A legal term
- B. Definition—engaging another person in sexual intercourse through the use of force and without the consent of the sexual partner
- C. Statutory rape—the act of sexual intercourse with a person under the age of legal consent. NOTE: sexual intercourse with a minor is rape, even with consent of the minor.
- D. Acquaintance rapes—involves someone known to the victim
- E. Victim not required by law to report it

F. Victim often receives no support from significant others
G. Victim often blamed by others
H. Nursing assessment
    1. Physical
        a. Last menstrual period
        b. Form of birth control used by client
        c. Determine last act of coitus before rape
        d. Penile penetration
        e. Orifices violated
        f. Duration of intercourse
        g. Use of condom by perpetrator
        h. Has client bathed, showered, douched, urinated, defecated, vomited, cleansed mouth?
        i. Pelvic exam
        j. Swabs taken of body cavities for semen
        k. Sleep disturbances
        l. Sobbing
        m. Crying
        n. Headaches
        o. Oropharyngeal trauma due to oral penetration
        p. Gastrointestinal disturbances
    2. Emotional
        a. Fear
        b. Loss of control
        c. Guilt for having survived
        d. Shame
        e. Embarrassment
        f. Humiliation
        g. Obsessive thoughts—what could have done differently
        h. Anger
        i. Revenge
        j. Change in residence
        k. Changes in relationships with men
        l. Hesitation to tell others for fear of not being believed
I. Nursing diagnoses
    1. Fear
    2. Anxiety
    3. Social isolation
    4. Body image disturbances
    5. Alteration in self-concept
    6. Alteration in mood
    7. Ineffective individual coping

     8. Alteration in comfort
     9. Sleep pattern disturbances
J. **Nursing interventions for the victim**
     1. Encourage not to shower, bathe, douche, or change clothing
     2. Preserve all evidence
     3. Treat physical injuries
     4. Reassure of safety
     5. Help victim refrain from self-blame
     6. Refer to crisis intervention, legal aid
     7. Refer to support groups

REVIEW QUESTIONS

1. A client exhibits a flushed face, muscle rigidity, and quickened body movements. These characteristics most likely reflect
   a. A tendency toward violence
   b. Characteristics of anger
   c. Manifestations of aggression
   d. Feelings of annoyance

2. The registered nurse is discussing with a student the guidelines for the use of restraints. Which of the statements by the student indicates a need for clarification?
   a. An adequate number of staff are needed before restraints are attempted
   b. Being restrained may help a client gain physical control
   c. A physician's order is required initially, followed by frequent renewal
   d. The use of restraints requires the supervision of a licensed and certified professional

3. A spouse comes into the health clinic having experienced family violence as a victim. Which group of client characteristics are anticipated by the nurse as the initial interview proceeds?
   a. Self-absorption, suspicious, perception of people as property
   b. Low self-esteem, dependent, perception of being captive in the system
   c. Family dysfunction, impermeable boundaries to outsiders, lack of trust
   d. Absence of humor, lack of flexibility, deficiency of intimacy

4. In a crisis center the nurse interacts with many victims of violence. To best meet these victims' needs the nurse must identify that the cycle of violence in relationships follows the sequence of
   a. Honeymoon period, tension-building phase, explosion
   b. Explosion, truce, honeymoon period
   c. Tension-building phase, explosion, honeymoon phase
   d. Verbal assaults, lack of control, truce

5. Which is least urgent in the initial interaction with a victim of rape?
   a. Preservation of all evidence
   b. Establishment of a trusting professional-client relationship
   c. Provision of referrals to a crisis intervention, legal aid center
   d. Provision of physical and emotional safety

ANSWERS, RATIONALES, AND TEST-TAKING TIPS

Rationales	Test-Taking Tips

1. **Correct answer: b**

   These are characteristics of anger. In option *a*, violence is a physical force that arouses fear in others to the point that their personal safety is threatened. Aggression is a learned reaction in which a motivating force, impulses, and feelings are converted into action. Feelings of annoyance may be part of the development of anger.

   The clues in the stem are the description of physical characteristics. Eliminate option *d*, which is "feelings." Eliminate option *c* since *manifestations of* typically is associated with *results,* as written there is not enough information to lead you to this conclusion. With knowledge that violence ends in the trauma of another person, eliminate option *a* because there is no victim given in the stem.

2. **Correct answer: d**

   The supervision of a registered nurse is required for the use of restraints. There is no certification for such interventions. The other options are correct statements.

   The best approach to this type of question is to read it slowly and carefully, since it is asking for an incorrect statement. After you have made a selection, reread the question and then read your choice to validate it.

3. **Correct answer: b**

   Option *a* describes characteristics of the abuser. Option *c* describes characteristics of the family in which there is an abuser and victims. Option *d* provides factors found in the family system of victimizers and victims.

   Note the clues in the stem for *client characteristics* and the time frame of the initial interview.

4. **Correct answer: c**

   The other choices are not in the proper sequence. Option *d*

   The question is asking for general phases, so eliminate option d.

provides specific factors that might be found within each part of the cycle.

Of the remaining options, use common sense to realize that situations first build, then burst, followed by a honeymoon phase of love, tenderness and truce. The cycle then repeats.

5. **Correct answer: c**

Referrals are typically done last, before discharge.

The clue in the stem is the time element—the initial interaction with the client. Referrals are implemented toward the end of the interaction with the client in the emergency unit.

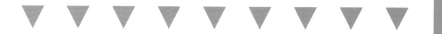

Affective Disorders

CHAPTER 13

STUDY OUTCOMES

After completing this chapter, the reader will be able to do the following:

▼ Define mood and varying levels of mood disorder.

▼ Describe the concepts of grief, depression, and mania.

▼ Discuss predisposing and precipitating factors in the development of mood disorders.

▼ Assess clients for suicide risk and plan interventions to provide safety.

▼ Apply the nursing process to the client experiencing a mood disorder.

KEY TERMS

Anhedonia	Loss of pleasure in activities of interest in the past.
Grief	Normal subjective response to loss.
Hypomania	Lower level of mania.
Mania	Mood that is elevated, expansive, irritable, and/or hyperactive.
Mood	Prolonged emotional state that influences one's whole personality and life functioning.
Object loss	Traumatic separation of a person from significant object of attachment.
Psychomotor agitation	Restlessness and speeded up body processes.
Psychomotor retardation	Slowing down of body process.
Suicidal attempt	Person believes that his/her self-destructive act will cause his/her death.
Suicidal gesture	Act of self-harm that is not necessarily life threatening.
Suicidal ideation	Thoughts of killing oneself.
Suicidal threat	Verbalization of wish to kill oneself.
Suicide	Intentional action taken to end one's own life.
Vegetative symptoms	Manifested by sleep disorders, eating disorders, weight loss, constipation, anhedonia.

CONTENT REVIEW

I. Mood disorders
A. Definition—mood or affective disturbance that affects behavior
B. Abnormal elaboration of sadness and grief
C. Oldest psychiatric illness
D. Maladaptive in nature
E. Incapacitating in nature
F. Ten theories as to cause of mood disorders
   1. Neurochemistry theory
      a. Catecholamine—deficiency of norepinephrine
      b. Serotonin decreased
      c. Monoamine oxidase inhibitors, used as a treatment for mood disorders, increase secretion of both norepinephrine and serotonin
   2. Hormonal theory
      a. Hypersecretion of cortisol
      b. Dexamethasone suppression test supports this hypersecretion (Box 13-1)

Box 13-1. Dexamethasone Suppression Test

In a subgroup of depressed clients, a disinhibition or lack of inhibition of plasma cortisol exists

The Test

1. The client receives 1 mg of dexamethasone by mouth at 11 P.M.
2. The client receives a barbiturate to ensure adequate sleep
3. At 8:00 the following morning, the client's cortisol level is determined. The level will be depressed.
4. At 4:00 the same afternoon, the client's cortisol level is determined. The afternoon level will be elevated. This is an abnormal finding, as the level should remain depressed for 24 hours after administration of the dexamethasone. This indicates a disinhibition or lack of inhibition of plasma cortisol. The abnormal finding of depressed clients.

From Stuart G and Sundeen S: *Principles and practices of psychiatric nursing,* ed 4, St Louis, 1991, Mosby.

3. Biological rhythms
   a. Circadian rhythm disturbance (early-morning awakening)
   b. Decreased total sleep time
   c. Increased dream time
   d. Difficulty falling asleep
   e. Decreased rapid eye movement (REM) sleep
4. Defects in immune system
5. Genetics
6. Psychoanalytical theory
   a. Response to loss
   b. Anger is turned inward on self
   c. Ineffective grieving results in depression
   d. Loss of self-esteem
   e. Helplessness
   f. Powerlessness
   g. Trauma in oral phase—need for warmth, affection, and appreciation
7. Behavioral theory
   a. Fail to receive positive reinforcement
   b. Learned helplessness—Seligman
      (1) No control over situations
      (2) Neither you nor anyone else can do anything
      (3) Negative expectations
   c. Object loss
      (1) Loss during childhood predisposes to depression

(2) Correlation between the onset of depression and disappointment in love relationships

(3) Repetition of childhood loss of a love object

(4) Early traumatic experience is predisposer to later depressions following any loss

(5) Disappointment occurs before Oedipal stage, when libido is still narcissistic: love object is treated as part of self, so loss involves part of self

(6) Result of inadequate mothering or loss of mother through various ways such as her going to work, going on vacation, or becoming ill

8. Cognitive—Beck theory
   a. Altered way of thinking
   b. Negative expectations
   c. Cognitive triad
      (1) Negative perception of self
      (2) Negative interpretation of experiences
      (3) Negative view of the future
   d. Obstacles to goals are present
   e. Self is helpless
   f. Control over life is hopeless

9. Sociological theory
   a. Loss of power
   b. Loss of status
   c. Loss of identity

10. Holistic-Integrated theory
    a. Genetic
    b. Biological
    c. Psychoanalytical
    d. Behavioral
    e. Cognitive
    f. Sociological

G. **Five types of precipitating events**
   1. Loss
      a. Real or imagined
      b. Person, status, self-esteem, body part or function
      c. Symbolic meaning—makes it difficult to understand. Example: moving to new home means loss of friends, memories, neighbors.
      d. Loss of hope
      e. Need to understand earlier losses and their resolutions

    f. Grief complicated by
      (1) Unresolved past losses
      (2) Ambivalent feelings
      (3) Uncertainty of loss, such as when someone is kidnapped or missing in action
      (4) Cultural denial, such as when one is expected to be the strong one
      (5) Lack of support from significant other

2. Major life events
    a. Interpersonal conflict
    b. Disruption of life patterns
    c. Exit or entrance of significant persons, such as when a child goes to college or there is a new stepmother

3. Roles
    a. Stressful social roles
    b. Neighborhood
    c. Job
    d. Financial affairs
    e. Homemaking
    f. Parenting
    g. Marriage/divorce
    h. Unemployment
    i. Retirement

4. Coping skills/support systems
    a. Socioeconomic status
    b. Families
    c. Interpersonal relationships

5. Physical changes
    a. Drug-induced depressions
      (1) Antihypertensives
      (2) Amphetamines
      (3) Alcohol
      (4) Barbiturates
    b. Medical illnesses
      (1) Viruses
      (2) Nutritional problems
      (3) Endocrine disorders
      (4) Blood dyscrasias
      (5) Multiple sclerosis
      (6) Tumors
      (7) Cerebrovascular disease
    c. Chronic debilitating illness

II. Epidemiology and treatment of mood disorders

    A. Incidence of depression

        1. Major depression—10% of all depressions

        2. 15 to 30% of all adults experience clinical depressive episodes

        3. 25% of persons with depressive symptoms seek professional mental health attention

        4. 50 to 80% of suicides are attributed to depression

        5. 75% of psychiatric hospitalizations are related to depression

    B. Prevalence of depression

        1. Women to men—2:1

        2. One third of medical inpatients report mild to moderate depression

    C. Incidence of mania

        1. 0.6 to 0.88% of U.S. adult population

        2. Higher incidence in women than men

        3. People under 50 are at higher risk of a first attack (Stuart and Sundeen, 1995)

    D. Effective treatment modalities

        1. Electroconvulsive therapy

        2. Antidepressant drugs

            a. Tricyclics

            b. Monamine oxidase inhibitors

            c. Seratonin reuptake inhibitors

        3. Antimania drugs

            a. Lithium preparations

            b. Anticonvulsants

                (1) Tegretol (Carbamazepine)

                (2) Depakene, myproic acid (Valproate)

        4. Individual psychotherapy

        5. Group psychotherapy

        6. Family therapy

        7. Cognitive therapy

            a. Increases self-esteem

            b. Modifies negative expectations

            c. Increases sense of control over goals and expectations

III. Three Levels of depression

    A. Mild depression

        1. Transitory—lasting less than 2 weeks (usually 1 or 2 days)

        2. Triggered by external events

            a. Loss

            b. Failing a test

            c. Not getting a promotion

3. Experience follows normal grief reaction
4. Assessment findings (most common to least common)
   a. Feel blue
   b. Sad
   c. "Down in the dumps"
   d. Let down or disappointed
   e. Mild alterations in sleep patterns
      (1) Not enough sleep
      (2) Always tired
   f. May feel less alert
   g. May increase use of alcohol or drugs
   h. Irritability
   i. Uninterested in spending time with others

B. **Moderate depression (dysthymia)**
   1. Experience a sense of change
   2. Persists over time
   3. Often seek help
   4. Assessment findings (lowest impairment to greatest impairment)
      a. Despondent
      b. Dejected
      c. Gloomy
      d. Low self-esteem
      e. Powerlessness
      f. Helplessness
      g. Ineffectiveness
      h. May experience intense anxiety and anger
      i. Diurnal variation—may feel better at certain time of day, such as morning
      j. Does not experience pleasure
      k. Thoughts are slow
      l. Difficulty concentrating
      m. Rumination
      n. Negative thinking
      o. Suicidal thoughts
      p. Social withdrawal
      q. Irritability
      r. Poor hygiene
      s. Psychomotor retardation or agitation
      t. Increased use of alcohol or drugs
      u. Somatic complaints
         (1) Headache
         (2) Chest pain

(3) Back pain
(4) Indigestion
(5) Nausea
(6) Vomiting
(7) Constipation
v. Anorexia
w. Weight loss
x. Fatigue
y. Menstrual changes
z. Sleep disturbances
(1) Initial insomnia—client has trouble falling asleep
(2) Middle insomnia—client has no difficulty falling asleep; wakes up in the middle of the night and, with difficulty, is able to return to sleep

C. **Severe depression (major depression)**
1. Intense
2. Pervasive
3. May or may not be psychotic
4. Assessment findings (lowest impairment to greatest impairment) (Clinical Example 13-1)
a. Despair
b. Hopelessness
c. Flat affect
d. Worthlessness
e. Guilt
f. Self-destructive thoughts
(1) Wishes to die
(2) May lack energy to act on thought

Clinical Example 13-1. Severe Depression

Client is a 72-year-old married woman admitted with severe recurrent affective disorder since the age of 35. She has shown a progressive 2-month deterioration, manifested by withdrawal from usual social activities, agitation, feelings of hopelessness, extreme fatigue, insomnia manifested by 2 hours each night of uninterrupted sleep, poor concentration (cannot read a page in a book), and anorexia with a 20-pound weight loss in 2 months. Client was unable to attend any social functions outside of her home and displayed so much anxiety that she was unable to sit long enough to have her hair done at her hairdresser's. She was treated with tricyclic antidepressants, family therapy with her husband and children, and electroconvulsive therapy. After 5 ECT treatments and 2 weeks of tricyclic therapy, the client was markedly improved, returned to her usual level of functioning, and returned home.

    g. Delusions reflect
        (1) Worthlessness—"My brain is full of maggots"
        (2) Guilt—"I've been sent to the penitentiary for life"
        (3) Powerlessness—"Someone is controlling my
             thoughts"
    h. Hallucinations
    i. Severe psychomotor retardation
        (1) All movement may stop
        (2) Robotlike in appearance
    j. Agitated pacing or walking
        (1) Pulling hair
        (2) Rubbing skin or hair
    k. Poor posture
        (1) Slumping
        (2) Curling up—fetal position
    l. Decreased speech—described as "poverty of speech"
    m. Disheveled, unkempt appearance
    n. Social withdrawal
    o. Poor concentration
    p. Overwhelmed by simple tasks
    q. Constipation
    r. Urinary retention
    s. Lack of sexual interest—impotence
    t. Marked loss of weight
    u. Anorexia
  *v. Sleep disturbances—terminal insomnia most common;
      client has no difficulty falling asleep, but has early-morning
      awakening without being able to return to sleep
  *w. Diurnal variation—feels worse in morning and better as
      day goes on
  *These findings are most helpful to differentiate between the
  levels of depression

IV. Application of the nursing process with the depressed client

  A. **Nursing assessment**
    1. Tools for measuring levels of depression
      a. Beck's Depression Inventory—measures feelings and
        behavior demonstrated by the depressed person
      b. Zung's Self-Rated Depression Scale—measures the level
        and pervasiveness of depression
      c. Miller Hope Scale—measures 11 critical elements of hope

2. Areas of assessment
   a. Sleep pattern
   b. Appetite
   c. Suicidal thoughts
   d. Activity level
   e. Affect
   f. Cognition
      (1) Cognitive triad
      (2) Attention span
   g. Orientation
      (1) Hallucinations
      (2) Delusions
   h. Toileting
   i. Weight
   j. Mood
      (1) Hopelessness
      (2) Helplessness
   k. Self-esteem
   l. Presence of physical illness
   m. Interest in activity
   n. Frequency of contact with others
   o. Diurnal variation
3. Common nursing diagnoses
   a. Alteration in self-esteem
   b. Self-care deficit
   c. Hopelessness
   d. Alteration in mood
   e. Risk for violence
   f. Risk for self-directed violence
   g. Alteration in elimination
   h. Alteration in nutritional status
   i. Maladaptive individual coping
   j. Alteration in sleep-rest pattern
   k. Social isolation
4. Goals for the depressed client
   a. Will verbalize confidence in self
   b. Will be able to tend to activities of daily living
   c. Will verbalize a positive outlook for the future
   d. Will verbalize interest and enjoyment in daily activities
   e. Will not physically harm others
   f. Will not physically harm self
   g. Will return to a normal bowel and bladder routine

    h. Will eat a balanced diet
    i. Will effectively cope with life stressors without high levels of anxiety or sadness
    j. Will return to normal sleep patterns present before the depression
    k. Will engage in social relationships with others
5. Nursing interventions with the depressed client
    a. Encourage client to discuss recent losses or changes in life situation
    b. Encourage client to express sadness and anger
    c. Encourage assertiveness training
    d. Encourage daily exercise
    e. Assist with ADLs if client unable
    f. Ensure adequate nutrition and sleep
    g. Assess for suicidal thoughts and intervene to provide safety as necessary
    h. Relieve physical complaints
    i. Allow adequate time for verbal responses
    j. Do not leave alone for extended periods
    k. Encourage use of the problem-solving approach
    l. Emphasize positive thinking
    m. Do not use an overly cheerful approach—makes them sadder
    n. Encourage participation in group activities
    o. Provide activities for easy mastery to increase self-esteem, such as cleaning off tables
    p. Limit decision making
    q. Provide tasks to help alleviate guilt, such as folding laundry, cleaning tables, washing windows
    r. Provide information about diagnosis, medications, and treatment of depression
    s. Help develop short-term goals
6. Medical treatment of depressed client
    a. Antidepressant medications
    b. Electroconvulsive therapy
7. Evaluation questions
    a. Is mood more animated?
    b. Does client report feeling better about self?
    c. Does client report pleasure in life?
    d. Has activity level increased or decreased?
    e. Has negative thinking decreased?
    f. Does client state he/she is no longer harmful to self?
    g. Does client initiate new friendships or reestablish old ones?

V. Suicidal behavior

A. Definition—intentional action taken to end one's life

B. Two theories as to the cause of suicidal behavior

   1. Psychoanalytical theory

      a. Eros—instinct for life

      b. Thanatos—instinct for death

      c. Thanatos is present in all

      d. Ambivalence in suicidal clients—results of conflict of eros and thanatos

      e. Anger turned inward—kills self instead of object he/she wishes to destroy

      f. Stressful life events activate the death wish

   2. Sociological theory

      a. Relationship between social conditions and incidence of suicide

      b. Durkheim—four forms of suicide

         (1) Egoistic—lacks group support; results in extreme individualism

         (2) Altruistic—identifies strongly with group; willing to die for group's ideas and purposes

         (3) Anomic—period of normlessness; society undergoes changes

         (4) Fatalistic—excessive regulation; opposite of anomic

      c. Farberon

         (1) Religion

         (2) Legal sanctions

         (3) Philosophical beliefs

         (Modified from Rawlins et al, 1993)

C. High-risk groups for suicidal behavior (all of these groups are at risk for suicide and should be assessed as such)

   1. Substance abusers

   2. Police

   3. Physicians

   4. Previous attempters

   5. Adolescents

   6. Terminally ill

   7. Older adults

   8. Accident-prone

   9. Certain minority groups

  10. Psychotic clients

  11. Medically ignored clients (illness not validated)

  12. Depressed clients

13. People who have experienced a loss of an important person early in life (death trend)
14. Eating-disordered
15. Disabled
16. Religious cults

D. **Myths related to suicide**
1. One should not take a suicide threat as serious
2. It is harmful to discuss suicide with a client
3. Only psychotic people commit suicide
4. People who talk about it will not do it
5. A failed suicide attempt should be treated as manipulative behavior
6. Suicide occurs only in lower socioeconomic levels

E. **Clues to suicide—behaviors to watch**
1. Giving away prized possessions
2. Making out or changing a will
3. Taking out or adding to insurance policies
4. Cancelling social engagements
5. Any change in behavior, positive or negative
6. Sleep difficulties
7. Feelings of hopelessness
8. Difficulty in concentrating
9. Loss of interest in friends, work, school, activities

F. **Dynamics underlying suicidal behavior**
1. Ambivalence
   a. Struggle between self-preserving and self-destructive forces
   b. Threaten or attempt suicide, then try to be rescued
2. Guilt
   a. Pervasive sense of being wrong or having done something wrong
   b. Guilt feeling exaggerated
   c. Feel responsible for all failures and wrongs
   d. Feel sinful
3. Anger and aggression
   a. Aggression turned inward
   b. Manipulative behavior—uses threats of suicide to control others
   c. Physical neglect or risk-taking behavior
4. Helplessness and hopelessness
   a. Life is hopeless
   b. Self is helpless
   c. No meaning or purpose to life

   5. Loneliness
      a. Emptiness
      b. Feel lonely even when others present
   6. Future orientation
      a. No sense of the future
      b. Unable to visualize death
   7. Reunion fantasy
      a. Life after death
      b. Rejoining with deceased loved ones
 G. **Application of the nursing process with the suicidal client**
   1. Nursing assessment
      a. Do they have a plan?
         (1) What is it?
         (2) How lethal?
         (3) How likely is death to occur? (Table 13-1)
         (4) Do they have the means to carry out the plan? For example, do they have a gun?
      b. History of attempts
         (1) Attempted before?
         (2) Lethality?
         (3) What was outcome?
         (4) Was the client accidentally rescued?
         (5) Have the past methods been the same, or have methods increased in lethality?
      c. Connection to others
         (1) Is the client alone?
         (2) Is the client alienated from others?
         (3) Are significant others giving negative messages to the client?

Table 13-1. Suicide Lethality

Low Lethality	High Lethality
Gas in house	Carbon monoxide poisoning
Cutting wrists	High doses of Aspirin and Tylenol
Some antianxiety agents (example: Valium)	Tricyclic antidepressants
	Shooting
Over-the-counter drugs excluding aspirin and Tylenol	Jumping
	Hanging
	Drowning
	Barbiturates
	Vehicular accidents
	Exposing oneself to extreme cold

    d. Presence of hostility

    e. Presence of hallucinations, such as voices telling them to kill themselves

    f. Presence of substance abuse

    g. Any recent losses

    h. Presence of physical illness

    i. Changes in behavior

    j. Presence of depression

    k. Any environmental changes

        (1) Family discord

        (2) A move of household or job

        (3) Unemployment

        (4) Retirement

        (5) Child's going away to college or moving back home

2. Client goals

    a. Client will not harm self

    b. Client will exhibit an absence of suicidal thoughts, gestures, comments

3. Nursing diagnosis—Risk for self-directed violence

4. Nursing planning and interventions

    a. Remove from danger by confiscating sharp objects, pills, other harmful objects

    b. Do not leave alone

    c. Remove to a physically safe environment

    d. Assume a nonjudgmental, caring attitude

    e. Organize a plan with client

        (1) Contract

        (2) Written, dated, and signed

        (3) Indicate alternative behavior at times of suicidal thoughts

    f. Keep active in daily activity—assign simple tasks

    g. Connect client with family, especially if client is

        (1) Confused

        (2) Angry

        (3) Uninterested

    h. Check that visitors do not leave harmful objects in client's room

    i. Do not allow client to leave the unit for tests or procedures unless accompanied by staff

5. Evaluation questions

    a. Does the client have more effective coping strategies for dealing with stress?

      b. Has the client remained free from suicidal ideation, threats, or gestures?

      c. Is client aware of community resources for help, such as the crisis phone line?

VI. Bipolar disorder

  A. DSM IV categories

    1. Bipolar I disorder—one or more manic or mixed episodes, usually accompanied by a major aggressive episode

    2. Bipolar II disorder—one or more major depressive episodes with one hypomanic episode

    3. Cyclothymia—numerous periods of hypomanic symptoms that do not meet the criteria for a manic episode, and numerous periods of depression that do not meet the criteria for a major depression

  B. Characterized by episodes of mania and depression

  C. Mania is a response to depression

  D. Levels of mania and depression are equivalent

  E. Three theories of causality

    1. Genetic

      a. Family history of depression

      b. Family history of mania

    2. Biological

      a. Increased norepinephrine and serotonin

      b. Chromosomal abnormalities

      c. Disruption in circadian rhythms

      d. EEG changes

      e. Heat trauma

      f. Drug-induced, as with anticonvulsants

    3. Psychoanalytical

      a. Loss, real or imagined, precipitates depression

      b. Mania defends against depression

      c. Anxiety and tension are denied and result in elated behavior

  F. Nursing assessment and findings of three levels of mania

    1. Hypomania

      a. Happy-go-lucky

      b. Extroverted

      c. Life of the party

      d. Confident

      e. Uninhibited

      f. Easily becomes irritable

      g. Free of worry
      h. Unconcerned with feelings of others
      i. Moves quickly from one subject to another
      j. Decreased ability to concentrate
      k. Exaggerated sense of importance
      l. Increased distractibility
      m. Increased motor activity
      n. "Catchy" euphoria—the observer begins to experience the euphoria
      o. Increased sex drive
      p. Engages in superficial relationships

2. Mania
      a. Affect is "high"
      b. Expansive
      c. Becomes angry quickly
      d. Unstable affect
      e. Flight of ideas—sudden, continuous shifts in topics
      f. Pressure of speech
      g. Grandiose and persecutory delusions
      h. Inappropriate dress
          (1) Excessive makeup
          (2) Too much jewelry
          (3) Brightly colored, poorly matched outfits
          (4) Inappropriate for weather, setting
          (5) Bizarre outfits
      i. Motor activity urgent
          (1) Meddles in the business of others
          (2) Rearranges furniture
          (3) Makes and remakes beds
          (4) Frequently changes clothing
          (5) Spends money
          (6) Risky driving
          (7) Increased interest in formal education
      j. Little or no appetite
      k. Days with no sleep
      l. Exhausted yet still active
      m. Sexually promiscuous
      n. Environmental stimuli distracts attention

3. Delirium
      a. Extreme excitement, elation, anger
      b. Disoriented
      c. Incoherent, uses new words

        d. Agitated, gesturing
        e. May injure self or others with frantic activity
        g. Grandiose or religious delusions
        h. Exhaustion
        i. Possible death
        j. Disheveled
        k. Poor hygiene

G. Application of the nursing process with the manic client

  1. Nursing assessment
      a. Motor activity
      b. Sleep-rest pattern
      c. Nutritional status
      d. Appearance
      e. Mood
      f. Thought process
      g. Thought content
      h. Self-esteem

  2. Nursing diagnoses
      a. Alteration in self-esteem
      b. Alteration in sleep-rest pattern
      c. Alteration in thought processes
      d. Alteration in nutritional status
      e. Alteration in fluid or electrolyte balance
      f. Alteration in interpersonal relationships

  3. Client goals
      a. Client will have adequate sleep/rest
      b. Client will have well-balanced diet
      c. Client will not experience delusions or hallucinations
      d. Client will have fluid and electrolyte balance within normal limits
      e. Client will establish meaningful interpersonal relationships
      f. Client will comply with medication regime (see Chapter 6, p. 110)

  4. Nursing interventions
      a. Set limits on inappropriate behaviors
      b. Reduce environmental stimuli
      c. Supervise administration of medications
      d. Ensure adequate nutrition and sleep—finger foods available throughout the day
      e. Help client focus on one topic during conversation
      f. Ignore or distract client from grandiose thinking
      g. Present reality

        h. Have consistent nurse assigned to care for client
        i. Dispense ordered medications
            (1) Carbamazepine (Tegretol)
            (2) Lithium (Eskalith)
        j. Provide information about diagnoses, medications, and treatment
        k. Promote a realistic self-esteem
        l. Use calm, slow interactions
        (Modified from Rawlins et al, 1993)

5. Evaluation criteria: Does the client have
    a. Adequate sleep/rest?
    b. Adequate nutrition?
    c. Fluid and electrolyte balance within normal limits?
    d. Realistic self-perception?
    e. Absence of a thought disorder?
    f. Meaningful interpersonal relationships?
    g. Compliance with medications?

REVIEW QUESTIONS

1. In assessing the needs of a depressed client admitted for an attempted overdose, the nurse would
   a. Encourage the client in a cheerful approach
   b. Keep the client busy to distract the client from suicidal thoughts
   c. Question the client about present suicidal thoughts
   d. Make plans for discharge to avoid depression at home

2. The nurse's primary responsibility in caring for a severely depressed client who is feeling better is to
   a. Protect the client from self-harm
   b. Reassure the client of the goals of the therapy
   c. Encourage adequate nutritional intake
   d. Obtain more personal information about the client

3. According to the dynamics of suicide, persons who feel isolated, hopeless, and helpless use the attempt of suicide to
   a. Make others feel remorse over their relationship with the suicidal individual
   b. Communicate a final message to others
   c. Hasten their passage to a better world
   d. Relate that they perceive suicide as the only available option

4. An appropriate nursing diagnosis of a client with a major depression is
   a. Alteration in activity
   b. Alteration in perceptions
   c. Alteration in affect
   d. Alteration in social activity

5. A client has been admitted to the mental health unit with a diagnosis of bipolar disorder. During assessment of the client's emotional status, which statement should the nurse expect the client to make when asked if the client is concerned about the family?
   a. "Why should I be worried?"
   b. "I hope they're okay"
   c. "I'm a failure as a person"
   d. "I'm worried about their welfare"

ANSWERS, RATIONALES, AND TEST-TAKING TIPS

Rationales	Test-Taking Tips

1. **Correct answer: c**

   The client was admitted with an attempted overdose. It is important to question the client about current suicidal ideation, then take the appropriate interventions.

   Read the question carefully to identify that the focus is for assessment of the client. The only assessment activity in the options is *c*.

2. **Correct answer: a**

   Appropriate precautions must always be considered. Client safety is always the nurse's first priority. When the depressed client is feeling better, the risk of suicide is the greatest, since at this time the client has more energy than during the severe depression.

   All of the responses are correct. The question is asking for the primary responsibility. Safety and confidentiality of clients are the two priority concerns in any given situation.

3. **Correct answer: d**

   Clients who are suicidal are not able to see any other available options. They have decreased levels of coping, and they view suicide as their only alternative to resolve their problems.

   Options *a, b,* and *c* may be reasons given in suicidal notes. However, the act of suicide is taken when no other alternatives are seen. Note that the question is asking about the dynamics of suicide, not about what might be written on a note.

4. **Correct answer: c**

   Depressed clients display little interest in themselves, others, or their surroundings. They display quiet, withdrawn behavior, with little socialization.

   Affect is a feeling, tone, or mood. The nursing diagnosis in option *c* best represents the depressed client's demeanor. The other diagnoses may be appropriate but are not the best choice, since they only address one aspect of a depressed client's overall behavior.

5. Correct answer: a

Clients with bipolar disorder experience elevated self-esteem, grandiose thinking, power, and self-importance. They have little or no concern for others during the manic phase of this disorder.

If you have no idea of the correct answer, cluster the three responses with the "I" statements and select option *a*.

▼ ▼ ▼ ▼ ▼ ▼ ▼ ▼ ▼ ▼   ▼ ▼ ▼

Psychotic Disorders

STUDY OUTCOMES

After completing this chapter, the reader will be able to do the following:

▼ Discuss the sociocultural, biochemical, developmental, and psychodynamic factors that contribute to the development of schizophrenia.

▼ Discuss the assessment findings of schizophrenia in the areas of cognition, perception, motor behavior, and interpersonal relationships.

▼ Describe individual, family, and environmental patterns of interaction associated with schizophrenia.

▼ Discuss defining characteristics of the various types of schizophrenia.

▼ Apply the nursing process with the client experiencing schizophrenia.

▼ Describe the characteristics of other psychotic disorders, including schizophreniform, schizoaffective, brief reactive psychosis, and atypical psychosis.

KEY TERMS

Affect	Outward display of emotion.
Ambivalence	Experiencing two opposing feelings at the same time; leads to inaction.
Autism	Cognitive process that is subjective in nature and relies on a personal, illogical interpretation of reality.
Automatic obedience	Carry out requests for an action in a robotlike fashion.
Clang association	Repetition of words or phrases that sound similar, or the substitution of a word that sounds like the appropriate word.
Cognition	Mental processes involved in obtaining knowledge.
Delusions	False belief firmly maintained despite evidence to the contrary.
Derealization	Feeling of strangeness or unreality with respect to the environment.
Echolalia	Repetition of words or phrases of another person as soon as he/she stops speaking.
Extrapyramidal effects	Side effects of antipsychotic medications that affect the extrapyramidial system and include findings such as tremors, drooling, and altered gait.
Hallucination	False sensory perception without corresponding stimuli involving any of the senses.
Illusion	Misperception or misinterpretation of reality. There are stimuli present: for example, a cloud is perceived as a flying saucer.
Looseness of associations	Thoughts do not flow together in a logical, connected manner.
Neologism	Privately coined word having meaning only to the speaker; not consensually validated.
Perception	Response of sensory receptors to external stimuli.
Psychosis	Reality is perceived differently from the way in which a majority of people perceive it.
Schizophrenia	A group of mental disorders characterized by psychotic features, inability to trust others, disordered thought process, and disrupted interpersonal relationships.
Stereotypy	Persistent, repetitive movements, such as walking around in circles.

| Waxy flexibility | Maintain a certain body posture indefinitely unless moved, despite feeling uncomfortable. |
| Word salad | A jumble of words that appear to have no relationship to one another. |

CONTENT REVIEW

I. Theories of etiology of schizophrenia

A. Developmental factors

1. Healthy parent-child relationship must meet child's needs. Four elements required
   a. Mothering—one must accurately perceive the child's needs
   b. Must respect child's needs
   c. Must consistently satisfy child's needs
   d. Child must be seen as a person in his/her own right
2. Potentially unhealthy parent-child relationship
   a. Mothering—one perceives child's needs on basis of his/her own needs
   b. Attempts to satisfy these needs through the child
   c. Child's needs are not respected
   d. Child's needs are not consistently met
3. Lack of maternal attention to child's needs leads to child's lack of trust in the mother
4. Lack of consistent attention to child's needs may create a suspicious attitude in child toward others
5. Results of anxiety in the maternal-child relationship
   a. "Bad Me" self-concept. "I'm no good, which is why I'm treated badly."
   b. "Not Me" self-concept. "I'm treated so badly that I must separate from reality and create my own reality (psychosis)."
   c. Faulty personal identity
      (1) Child's efforts to become autonomous are not supported
      (2) Child does not engage in developmental process of individuation
      (3) Child remains fused with environment
      (4) Child is unaware of personal boundaries
      (5) Child is unaware of self as a separate entity

B. Family-supported interaction factors

1. Indirect communication patterns within family
2. Highly repressed emotion

    3. Overinvolvement of family members in each other's affairs—lack of boundaries

    4. Bateson's double-bind theory

       a. Child given two conflicting messages at the same time

       b. No-win situation

       c. "Damned if you do and damned if you don't." Example: parent asks child for a hug then pushes child away.

       d. Results of repeated exposure

          (1) Rage

          (2) Apathy

          (3) Ambivalence

          (4) Anxiety

    5. Pathological family interaction—Lidz

       a. Family skew

          (1) Outwardly harmonious

          (2) Intrusive, overprotective mother

          (3) Child cannot exist without her supervision

          (4) Mother opposes autonomy

          (5) Child fearful of being engulfed by man

          (6) Child believes neither he nor his mother can get along without each other

          (7) Father passive and feels excluded from family

       b. Schismatic family

          (1) Overt conflict between parents

          (2) Competition for loyalty of the child

          (3) Child tries to please both parents

          (4) Child is family scapegoat

          (5) Child *appears to* cause parental conflicts

          (6) Communication is confusing and distorted

          (7) Child represses feelings to fit into parents' expectations

C. Psychoanalytic factors

    1. Failure of ego to mediate between id drives and the reality of the ego

    2. Ego functions

       a. Undeveloped

       b. Weak

       c. Impaired

    3. Primitive thinking predominates

    4. High anxiety results in impaired ability to relate to others

    5. Prolonged and/or intense anxiety with limited coping results in psychosis

D. **Sociocultural factors**
  1. Divorce rate rising
  2. Family less stable
  3. Less contact between generations
  4. Stressors cause problems in development of family intimacy
E. **Biological factors**
  1. Higher incidence of schizophrenia in family members of schizophrenic parents
  2. Identical twins separated at birth—if one has schizophrenia, the other does 58% of the time
  3. Brain changes
     a. Atrophy with enlargement of ventricles
     b. Decrease in brain's gross weight
     c. Decreased volume in limbic structures
     d. Distorted size and shape of cells in cortical and limbic areas
  4. Biological and biochemical factors are supported the most by scientific evidence as a cause of schizophrenia
F. **Biochemical factors**
  1. Dopamine theory—excess of dopamine
     a. Increased production
     b. Increased release
     c. Increased number of dopamine receptors
  2. Norepinephrine theory—may be increase in norepinephrine production or release
  3. Indolamine hypothesis—defect in metabolism of serotonin: dopamine product in the synthesis of norepinephrine increases blood pressure and increases urinary output
  4. Gamma-aminobutyric acid (GABA)—amino acid that is the principal inhibitor of neurotransmitters in the central nervous system
     a. Relationship between GABA and dopamine
     b. Decreased GABA has been associated with increased dopamine
G. **Endocrine factors**
  1. Low levels of follicle-stimulating hormone (FSH)—FSH stimulates growth of follicle in ovary and spermatogenesis in the testis
  2. Low levels of luteinizing hormone (LH)—LH stimulates development of the corpus luteum, which secretes progesterone
  3. Low prolactin levels—prolactin stimulates breast development and formation of milk in pregnancy
  4. Hypothyroidism

H. **Viral hypothesis**
1. Viral infection is precursor
2. Some viruses cause psychotic symptoms (HIV)
3. Structural changes in brain similar to those from viral infections

II. Epidemiology and treatment of schizophrenia

A. **Prevalence—0.5 to 1% of population**
1. Occurs equally between men and women
2. Occurs in all socioeconomic levels
3. More common in lower socioeconomic levels
4. Clients exhibit relapse rates of 50% in first year and 70% in second year after hospitalization
(Haber et al, 1992)
B. **Onset**
1. Men—mid twenties
2. Women—late twenties
3. Abrupt or insidious
C. **Prognosis**
1. One third get better with treatment
2. One third get better without treatment
3. One third do not get better with or without treatment—becomes a chronic process
4. Better prognosis
    a. Acute onset
    b. Later age at onset
    c. Good premorbid adjustment
        (1) Interpersonal relationships
        (2) Work history
        (3) School
    d. Female
    e. Existence of precipitating stressors
    f. Associated mood disturbance
    g. Brief duration of active-phase symptoms
    h. Minimal residual symptoms
    (Modified from American Psychiatric Association, 1994)
D. **Treatment**
1. Antipsychotic medications
2. Reality orientation therapy
3. Noninsight-oriented psychotherapy
4. Music, art, and poetry therapy

III. Behaviors indicative of schizophrenia

A. **Physical appearance**
  1. Disheveled
  2. Unkempt
  3. Body image distortions—delusional
     a. Skull is flat
     b. Joints falling apart
     c. Body parts no longer in proportion
  4. Preoccupation with somatic complaints—more aware of body functions
     a. Breathing
     b. Heartbeat
  5. Neglects eating, sleeping, and elimination
  6. Unable to make eye contact
  7. Motor activity
     a. Too little
        (1) Catatonic
        (2) May be totally immobilized
        (3) Unable to respond to commands
        (4) Responds only to commands—automatic obedience
        (5) Waxy flexibility—maintain a certain body posture indefinitely unless moved, despite feeling uncomfortable
     b. Movements repetitive or stereotyped (stereotypy—persistent, repetitive movements, such as walking around in circles)
     c. Too much
        (1) Agitation
        (2) Pacing
        (3) Inability to sleep
        (4) Loss of appetite
        (5) Loss of weight
        (6) Impulsiveness
     d. Volition—unable to initiate activity; also known as anergia
B. **Emotional characteristics**
  1. Massive mistrust
  2. Experiences world as threatening and unsafe
  3. Feelings not easily interpreted
  4. Ambivalence (Table 14-1)
  5. Common feelings
     a. Negativism

Table 14-1. Some Behavioral Manifestations of Ambivalence

Behavior	Description	Example
Compulsive rituals	Attempts to solve conflicting feelings by constant, repetitive activity, which may be stereotyped or seem meaningless	John has difficulty leaving his room. He gets up from the chair, takes three steps forward then three steps backward, sits again, touches the bed, stands up, taps the window, sits down, taps his knee three times, and then gets up and begins to walk forward again.
Negativism	Attempts to avoid opposing feelings by refusing, either verbally or nonverbally, to participate	Elizabeth's response to any request is always no. She refuses to get out of bed in the morning or participate in any ward activities. Once engaged in a given activity, the effort to have her change the activity is equally problematic.
Overcompliance	Attempts to deny responsibility for any action by doing only what another exactly instructs	Harold agrees to play checkers but will not move the pieces unless someone sits beside him to tell him exactly which way to move them and where to place them

From Rawlins R, Williams S, Beck C: *Mental health-psychiatric nursing: A holistic life-cycle approach,* ed 3, St Louis, 1992, Mosby.

        b. Helplessness
        c. Decreased self-esteem
        d. Anxiety
        e. Fear
        f. Anger
        g. Guilt
        h. Depression
        i. Ambivalence
    6. Emotional instability
        a. Shift is extreme
        b. No precipitants
    7. Affective disturbances
        a. Flat affect
            (1) Intensity of emotion less than expected
            (2) No feelings communicated in verbal and nonverbal responses

      (3) Example: a girl talks about being mugged with no expression of feeling

  b. Inappropriate affect

      (1) Content of thought differs from emotional tone

      (2) Example: a man laughs as he talks about his wife just dying

  c. Thought process

      (1) Fragmentation of thoughts

      (2) Blocking—person abruptly stops talking

      (3) Loose associations

          (a) Thoughts do not logically connect

          (b) Transitions cannot be observed. Example: "I love to go swimming. Blue is my favorite color. I'm going to the store today."

          (c) Answers questions in a nonsensical way. Example: Q: "Could you tell me your name?" A: "I love to dance."

      (4) Autistic thinking

          (a) Regression to self-centered way of thinking like a child

          (b) Environment perceived in a totally self-centered way

          (c) Everything that happens relates directly to the person

          (d) Subjective interpretations

          (e) May make up own words (neologisms) and assign private, unshared meanings to experiences. Example: looks at a glass and smiles, then laughs.

      (5) Magical thinking

          (a) A form of autistic thinking

          (b) Equates thinking with doing. Example: "I wish my mother to die." Therefore, "She is dead."

      (6) Concrete thinking

          (a) Unable to conceptualize meaning in words or thoughts

          (b) Understanding based on context is lost, as well as the understanding of the context in which a word is used. For instance, "bear" and "bare" may seem the same.

          (c) Logical categories or abstractions of common qualities are lost. Example: Q: "How are a dog and a cat alike?" A: "They both have ears." or "Both are animals."

    (d) Interprets proverbs concretely. Example: "People in glass houses shouldn't throw stones." Interpretation "The glass will break."

    (e) Cannot organize facts logically

(7) Delusions

    (a) Fixed false beliefs

    (b) Help to meet needs, such as for identity. For instance, "I'm the Virgin Mary" meets need of increased self-esteem or sense of importance.

    (c) Function to alleviate anxiety

    (d) Based on an element of truth—"punctiform insight" (Clinical Example 14-1)

    (e) Reflect denial of own unacceptable physical traits

    (f) Types of delusions (Table 14-2)

    (g) Process of a delusion

        (i) Experience a feeling, such as "I don't like myself"

        (ii) Denial of feeling

        (iii) Projection—"He doesn't like me"

        (iv) Result

            ▼ Decreased anxiety as ownership for feeling has been projected

            ▼ Saved self-esteem

Clinical Example 14-1. Fixed Delusion Based on an Element of Truth—"Punctiform Insight"

A 67-year-old divorced man has experienced numerous admissions to psychiatric hospitals with a diagnosis of paranoid schizophrenia. Years ago he was a Catholic, married man serving overseas in the army during WWII. During this tenure, he had an affair with a woman. The knowledge of this affair was shared by a friend (George) in the military. After the war both men returned to the United States, never to see or contact each other again. The client's marriage deteriorated and ended in divorce. He experienced much guilt related to his affair, and over the years developed a delusion that George and company were out to get him. Wherever the client would go, this company would follow him and send men up through the ventilation system of whatever building he was in. These men would shoot and kill him with vapor. The only protection for the client was to wrap himself in aluminum foil.

Table 14-2. Types of Delusions with Examples

Type	Definition	Example
Ideas of reference	A person believes certain events, situations, or interactions are directly related to himself/herself	A 40-year-old man telephones the police to inform them that he sees two people standing in front of his house who must be talking about him. He requests that a squad car be dispatched to stop the people from loitering in front of his house, which would interfere with their ability to talk about him.
Delusions of persecution	A person believes he/she is being harassed, threatened, or persecuted by some powerful force. A person may be driven to act in drastic ways by such persecutory thoughts.	A 35-year-old unemployed bookkeeper has always led an isolated life, with few friends or recreational interests. She worked for a large corporation whose clerical staff was about to be unionized. Monica became convinced that the supervisors were harassing the employees, including her, because they had voted to become union members. She believed that she was being singled out and harassed by her supervisor, who was giving her the most difficult and heaviest workload of all the bookkeepers. Monica eventually involved the company officers, her family, and childhood teachers in her delusional system, thinking they were all involved in a conspiracy to punish her because she joined the union. She resigned from her job as a protest against the harassment she felt she was receiving. She did not keep in touch with her friends at work, nor did she return their calls. One day she was spotted by a security guard, hovering outside the building where she had worked. The guard heard her muttering something about a conspiracy as she bent to light a greasy rag with a match. She was hospitalized after

Continued.

Table 14-2. Types of Delusions with Examples—cont'd

Type	Definition	Example
Delusions of persecution —cont'd		she attempted arson. She was discharged from the hospital 2 months later, with little change in her delusions of persecution except that she was no longer driven to act on her delusion.
Delusions of grandeur	A person attaches special significance to his/her position in relation to others or the universe, or has an exaggerated sense of self-aggrandizement that has no basis in reality; for example, the belief that he/she is an important person, either living or dead, is related to such a person, or is influential in important affairs	A 45-year-old unmarried woman walked around carrying a bundle swaddled in a baby blanket. She said it contained the baby Jesus and that she was his mother, Mary. She refused to put the bundle down because she thought people, envious of her special position, were trying to kidnap her baby.
Somatic delusions	A person believes that his or her body is changing or responding in an unusual way, which has no basis in reality	A 50-year-old man had gallbladder surgery in a general hospital. Following the surgery he began to complain to his family that he was convinced other vital organs had also been removed at the time of surgery. He claimed that his stomach had been removed, which he viewed as punishment for not taking his physician's advice about losing weight.

From Haber J, et al: *Comprehensive psychiatric nursing,* ed 4, St Louis, 1992, Mosby.

   (h) Unacceptable thoughts, feelings, actions, wishes come from outside

   (i) May become systematized

    (i) Organized

    (ii) Logical

    (iii) Fixed delusion (see Clinical Example 14-1)

 8. Perceptual distortions

  a. Illusions

   (1) Misrepresentations or misinterpretations of reality

   (2) Brief, transitory experiences

  b. Hallucinations (Table 14-3)

   (1) Perceptions of objects, sensations, or images with no basis in reality

   (2) Involve any of the five senses

   (3) A response to severe anxiety

   (4) Meet needs not met in reality

   (5) Phases in the development of hallucinations

    (a) Anxiety—daydreams to decrease discomfort

    (b) Perceptual awareness increases "listening attitude"—waits to experience the sensation

    (c) Projects experience outward—experiences hallucination

    (d) Sense of security or comfort

    (e) Hallucination becomes

     (i) Uncomfortable

     (ii) Commanding

     (iii) Threatening

     (iv) Disparaging

    (f) Hallucinations control behavior

   (6) Most common hallucinations are auditory or visual

C. **Disturbances in language usage and communication in schizophrenia (Table 14-4)**

 1. Interaction with others is based on ability to exchange ideas and thoughts

 2. Disorders in communication affect this relationship

 3. Language disturbances are related to disorders in thought process

 4. Unable to organize language

 5. May develop private language

 6. A single word or phrase may represent the whole meaning of the conversation

 7. Clients may feel they have communicated adequately

Table 14-3. Types of Hallucinations with Examples

Type	Definition	Example
Auditory	Voices or sounds heard by the client but not by others and that do not relate to objective reality	A client heard music not heard by others
Command	A type of auditory hallucination in which voices demand that the person perform some action, often aggressive toward self or others	Randy heard a screaming voice insisting that he stick his arms with needles
Visual	Visual images or sensations experienced by the client; the client may see images of figures, objects, or events that may be grotesque, frightening, or comforting	Sylvie thinks she sees a door close out of the corner of her eye, when in fact the door remains open
Olfactory	Odors that appear to be coming from specific or unknown places	Julie states that she smells onions no matter where she goes
Gustatory	Tastes are experienced that have no basis in reality	Randy states that, whenever he is in a room full of people, he develops a burning sensation on his tongue
Tactile	Strange body sensations that may or may not be part of a delusional system. At times tactile hallucinations involve misperceptions about body parts. This type of hallucination is common in alcohol toxicity.	A client in alcohol withdrawal feels as if insects are crawling inside his body

From Haber J, et al: *Comprehensive psychiatric nursing,* ed 4, St Louis, 1992, Mosby.

Table 14-4. Common Language Patterns in Schizophrenia

Pattern	Definition	Example
Neologism	"New word" devised that has special meaning only to the client	*Raffity* was a word used by Sylvia to mean someone she could not trust
Echolalia	Repetition of words or phrases heard from another person	After the nurse asked Julie to take her medication, Julie repeated, "Medication, medication, medication"
Verbigeration	Purposeless repetition of words or phrases used by clients with chronic schizophrenia	For many days Randy repeated, "NASA goes to the moon. NASA goes to the moon."
Metonymic speech	Use of words with similar meanings interchangeably	A client may say, "Please pass the spoon," when the intended message is, "Please pass the fork"
Clang association	Repetition of words or phrases that are similar in sound but in no other way	A client might say, "I want to go on an outing to the park, lark, dark, bark"
Word salad	Form of speech in which words or phrases are connected meaninglessly	The client might say, "Baby, throw ocean blue"
Stilted language	Refers to an overly and inappropriately formal communication pattern, usually written, which seems artificial and intellectual	A client might say, "Good morning, Judy. It is an exceptionally bright and glorious day, and I will attempt to be fastidious in my appreciation of it"
Pressured speech	Speaking as if the words are being forced out quickly (reflects the client's racing thoughts)	"I need my medication. Please give it to me because it was due 10 minutes ago and I feel very anxious and upset, okay?"
Mutism	Absence of verbal speech	Susan sat in the corner of the day room sucking her thumb (reflects regression also) and would not respond verbally to any attempts at communication

From Haber J, et al: *Comprehensive psychiatric nursing,* ed 4, St Louis, 1992, Mosby.

IV. Bleuler's four A's of schizophrenia

A. Bleuler made the first effort to identify behaviors typical of schizophrenia

B. Bleuler identified four primary symptoms: "the four A's" of schizophrenia

C. These symptoms were necessary for the diagnosis

D. Four A's
   1. Affective disturbance
   2. Ambivalence
   3. Associative disturbance—looseness of associations
   4. Autism

V. Positive and negative schizophrenia

A. Positive symptoms of schizophrenia
   1. Excess or distortion of normal functions
   2. Delusions
   3. Hallucinations
   4. Disorganized speech
   5. Disorganized or catatonic behavior
      a. Marked decrease in reactivity to environment
      b. Stupor—complete unawareness of environment
      c. Catatonic negativism—resistance to instructions
      d. Catatonic excitement—purposeless, excessive motor activity

B. Negative symptoms of schizophrenia
   1. Flat affect
   2. Alogia—brief, empty verbal replies
   3. Avolition—inability to initiate and persist in activity

VI. Description of and types of schizophrenia

A. Findings last at least 6 months

B. At least 1 month of active symptoms

C. Basic intellectual functions intact

D. Lack of insight is common

E. 10% of individuals commit suicide

F. Onset occurs in late teens to mid thirties

G. Equal occurrence between men and women

H. Incidence between 0.5% and 1%

I. Onset may be abrupt or insidious

J. Prodromal phase
   1. Social withdrawal
   2. Lack of interest in school or work
   3. Deterioration in hygiene and grooming

    4. Outbursts of anger

    5. Unusual behavior

K. Types of schizophrenia

    1. Paranoid schizophrenia

       a. Delusions—persecutory or grandiose

       b. Auditory hallucinations

       c. Anxiety

       d. Anger

       e. Aloofness

       f. Persecutory themes

       g. Suicidal behavior

       h. Violence

       i. Prognosis: better for occupational functioning and independent living

    2. Disorganized schizophrenia

       a. Disorganized speech

       b. Disorganized behavior

       c. Flat or inappropriate affect

       d. Silliness and laughter unrelated to speech

       e. Inability to perform activities of daily living

       f. Stereotyped behaviors

       g. Grimacing

       h. Mannerisms

       i. Insidious onset

       j. Prognosis: poor

    3. Catatonic schizophrenia

       a. Marked psychomotor disturbance

       b. Immobility

       c. Waxy flexibility

       d. Stupor

       e. Excessive, purposeless motor activity

       f. Negativism—rigid posture

       g. Echolalia

       h. Stereotypy—stereotyped or repetitive behavior

       i. Automatic obedience

       j. Echopraxia (mimic body movements of others)

       k. Risks

          (1) Malnutrition

          (2) Exhaustion

          (3) Dehydration

          (4) Hyperpyrexia

       l. Prognosis: fair

4. Undifferentiated schizophrenia
   a. Delusions
   b. Hallucinations
   c. Disorganized speech
   d. Disorganized or catatonic behavior
   e. Negative symptoms
   f. Does not meet criteria for paranoid, disorganized, or catatonic schizophrenia
   g. Prognosis: fair
5. Residual schizophrenia
   a. Without positive symptoms
   b. Have been diagnosed as schizophrenic in the past
   c. Negative symptoms re-present
   d. Time limited between attacks
   e. Present for many years
   f. Prognosis: poor

VII. Application of the nursing process with the schizophrenic client

A. Nursing assessment
   1. Physical status
      a. Hydration
      b. Nutrition
      c. Intake and output
      d. Bowel movements
      e. Total system review—clients often unaware of or do not report symptoms, such as broken bones
      f. Increased or decreased physical activity
      g. Postural—waxy flexibility
   2. Safety
      a. Assess for suicide risk
      b. Hallucinations may command clients to kill themselves or others
      c. May be dangerous to self or others based on persecutory delusions or hallucinations
   3. Interpersonal relationships
      a. Do they have a support system?
      b. Do they have any friends?
      c. How comfortable are they in one-on-one relationships?
   4. Thought process assessment
      a. Loose associations
      b. Autistic thinking

       c. Blocking

       d. Concrete thinking

       e. Delusions

          (1) Content of delusion

          (2) Type of delusion

       f. Orientation

   5. Affect

       a. Flat

       b. Inappropriate

   6. Perceptual distortions

       a. Hallucinations

       b. Illusions

   7. Ambivalence

       a. Ask "Do you ever have trouble making a decision?"

       b. Ask "Do you often feel two different ways about a situation?"

   8. Tardive dyskinesia

   9. Regressive behavior

B. Nursing diagnoses

   1. Impaired social interaction

   2. Self-esteem disturbance

   3. Risk for self-harm

   4. Risk for violence

   5. Sleep pattern disturbance

   6. Personal identity disturbance

   7. Sensory-perceptual alteration

   8. Impaired verbal communication

   9. Ineffective individual coping

  10. Altered nutrition

  11. Altered thought process

C. Goals

   1. Maintain an adequate balance of rest, sleep, and activity

   2. Maintain an adequate balance of nutrition, hydration, and elimination

   3. Be free of injury

   4. Participate in therapeutic milieu

   5. Communicate effectively with others

   6. Establish contact with reality

   7. Express feelings in an acceptable manner

   8. Verbalize increased feelings of self-worth

   9. Identify strengths and weaknesses

  10. Comply with prescribed regimen

  11. Begin to trust others

D. **Nursing interventions**
1. Begin with one-on-one interactions and progress to small groups as tolerated
2. Spend time with client, even when he/she is unable to respond
3. Only make promises you can realistically keep
4. Establish a daily routine
5. Help client improve grooming—assist them but do not do for them
6. Help client accept as much responsibility for personal grooming as he/she can
7. Reorient to person, place, and time as indicated
8. Help client establish what is real and unreal
9. Stay with client if client is frightened
10. Be simple, direct, and concise when speaking
11. Reassure client that the environment is safe
12. Remove client from group situations if behavior is too bizarre, disturbing, or dangerous to others
13. Make contact on client's level of behavior; unconditional acceptance
14. Set realistic goals
15. Initially, do not offer choices to the client. Example: "It is time to eat." vs "Would you like to eat now?"
16. Gradually assist client in making own decisions
17. Be alert to physical needs
18. Administer antipsychotic medication as ordered
19. Set limits on client's behavior when he/she is unable to do so
20. Decrease excessive stimuli in the environment
21. Intervention guidelines for *active hallucinations*
    a. Be aware of hallucination cues
        (1) Intent listening for no reason
        (2) Talking to person not present
        (3) Muttering to self
        (4) Inappropriate laughter
    b. Decrease stimuli or move client to another area
    c. Avoid conveying that you are also experiencing the hallucination ("I do not hear a voice")
    d. Respond verbally to anything real that the client talks about
    e. Encourage client to make staff member aware of hallucinations
    f. If client appears to be hallucinating, attempt to engage his/her attention through a concrete activity
    g. *Avoid touching client*

      h. Provide easy-to-do activities

      i. Provide a structured environment with routine activities of daily living

      j. Monitor for signs of increasing fear, anxiety, or agitation and intervene early

      k. Intervene with one-on-one contact, seclusion, PRN medication as necessary

      l. Encourage expression of feelings

      m. Show acceptance of behavior; do not joke about or judge behavior

22. Intervention guidelines for delusions

      a. Recognize the delusions as the client's perception of the environment

      b. Do not argue with client or try to convince him/her that the delusions are false

      c. Interact on the basis of real things

      d. Never convey to client that you accept the delusion as reality

      e. Encourage client to ventilate feelings

      f. If client thinks food is poisoned or he/she is not worthy of the food, it may be necessary to alter normal routines, such as using packaged food or food from home

      g. Build client's self-esteem

         (1) Give positive feedback for successes

         (2) Recognize accomplishments

         (3) Use one-on-one activities first

23. Guide client to utilize alternate means to express feelings

      a. Music therapy

      b. Art therapy

      c. Journaling

E. Evaluation criteria for client

1. Has had adequate sleep

2. Has maintained an adequate balance of nutrition, hydration, and elimination

3. Has remained free of injury

4. Has an increased sense of worth

5. Has exhibited a decrease in hallucinations and delusions to a manageable level

6. Has verbalized feelings to staff as they occur

7. Has listed strengths and weaknesses

8. Has been able to interact coherently with peers and staff

9. Has been able to participate in ward activities

VIII. Schizophreniform disorder
   A. Illness lasts 1 to 6 months
   B. Impaired social or occupational functioning is not required
   C. If the impairment lasts longer than 6 months, it is schizophrenia
   D. One third recover within 6 months
   E. Remaining two thirds progress to schizophrenia or schizoaffective disorder
   F. Confusion is usually present
   G. Typically client had good social and occupational functioning before disorder
   H. Absence of flat affect

   (Modified from *Diagnostic and statistical manual of mental disorders*, 4th ed, American Psychiatric Association, 1994)

IX. Schizoaffective disorder
   A. Major depression or bipolar disorder concurrent with symptoms of schizophrenia
   B. Delusions or hallucinations
   C. Mood symptoms last throughout disorder
   D. Pervasive depressed mood
   E. Poor occupational functioning
   F. Decreased social contact
   G. Difficulties with self-care
   H. Suicide risk
   I. Onset in early adulthood

   (Modified from *Diagnostic and statistical manual of mental disorders*, 4th ed, American Psychiatric Association, 1994)

X. Brief psychotic disorder
   A. Sudden onset
   B. Delusions
   C. Hallucinations
   D. Disorganized or catatonic behavior
   E. Lasts 1 to 30 days
   F. Client returns to premorbid level of functioning
   G. Overwhelming confusion
   H. High risk of suicide
   I. Occurs in adolescence or early childhood

XI. Atypical psychotic disorder-psychotic symptoms (delusions, hallucinations, disorganized speech, disorganized or catatonic behavior), but does not meet criteria for a specific psychotic disorder

REVIEW QUESTIONS

1. A client, age 25, with schizophrenia is told about the unit routine and is taken to the assigned room. On the way the psychiatric technician asks the client what brought the client to the hospital. The client replies, "A bus." This is an example of
   a. Denial
   b. A hallucination
   c. A rational answer
   d. Concrete thinking

2. A client newly diagnosed with schizophreniform disorder tells the nurse that the CIA is looking for him and will kill him if they find him. The best response is what?
   a. "That's ridiculous. No one is going to hurt you"
   b. "The CIA isn't interested in people like you"
   c. "Why do you think the CIA wants to kill you?"
   d. "I find what you are saying hard to believe"

3. A client tilts his head to the side, stops talking in midsentence, and listens intently. The nurse recognizes that the client is likely experiencing
   a. Somatic delusions
   b. Catatonic stupor
   c. Auditory hallucinations
   d. Pseudoparkinsonism

4. A client is diagnosed with catatonic schizophrenia. Which is a highest priority nursing diagnosis?
   a. Noncompliance
   b. Impaired communication
   c. Ineffective coping
   d. Self-care deficit

5. On arrival for admission to a voluntary unit, a female client loudly announces, "Everyone kneel, you are in the presence of the Queen of England." This is
   a. A delusion of self-belief
   b. A delusion of self-appreciation
   c. A nihilistic delusion
   d. A delusion of grandeur

ANSWERS, RATIONALES, AND TEST-TAKING TIPS

Rationales	Test-Taking Tips

1. Correct answer: d

This is a classic example of concrete thinking, which is the client's inability to conceptualize meaning in words or thought. Understanding based on context is lost as well as the understanding on the context in which a word is used. For example the words, bear and bare may seem the same. Logical categories of common qualities are lost; for example: question "How are a dog and a cat alike? answer: "They both have ears." Also, with concrete thinking the client is not able to organize facts logically.

Use your common sense to eliminate option *a,* denial, option *b,* hallucination and option *c,* a rational answer.

2. Correct answer: d

This is a therapeutic communication technique, voicing doubt. It is suggesting doubt to the client while attempting to do reality orientation. The other responses are nontherapeutic, since options *a* and *b* are giving opinions and option *c* is inappropriately validating what the client has said.

Select the response that sounds the most professional, with a validation that the nurse heard what the client said but does not necessarily agree with the client.

3. Correct answer: c

Hallucinations can occur in all five senses. Auditory hallucinations are when the

The key word in the stem is "listens." It clues in to the selection of auditory hallucinations.

client is hearing voices. This is a sensory perception that does not result from an external stimulus occurring in a waking state. Pseudoparkinsonism is nonintention tremors, most commonly pill rolling. Catatonic stupor lasts longer than a few minutes and occurs when the client does not move. Somatic delusions are beliefs that one's body or parts are diseased or distorted.

4. Correct answer: d

With this diagnosis, the client is withdrawn, stuporous, and experiencing muscle rigidity. The client is unable to care for his/her needs, so this becomes the responsibility of the nurse.

Of the given choices, note that three are psychosocial, *a, b,* and *c.* Select the physiological option based on the use of Maslow's hierarchy of needs.

5. Correct answer: d

This delusion is a gross exaggeration of the client's self-importance, wealth, power, or talents. There are no delusions as referenced in the other options. Nihilistic ideas are thoughts of nonexistence and hopelessness.

Associate that persons with grandiose delusions make grand entrances or appearances when entering new environments.

Paranoid Disorders

STUDY OUTCOMES

After completing this chapter, the reader will be able to do the following:

▼ Discuss the psychodynamics involved in the development of paranoid disorders.

▼ Describe the behavioral characteristics of the client experiencing a paranoid disorder.

▼ Describe the various types of paranoid disorders.

▼ Apply the nursing process with a client experiencing a paranoid disorder.

KEY TERMS

Grandiose delusion	False belief related to being famous, important, or wealthy.
Hypervigilance	A persistent sense of danger, which involves physiological arousal and heightened attention to the environment while in search of early warning signs of impending danger (Haber et al, 1992).
Paranoia	A behavioral manifestation representative of the defense mechanism of projection, whereby the person attributes his/her thoughts and impulses to others; a feeling of extreme suspicion (Stuart and Sundeen, 1995).
Paranoid delusion	The false belief that one is being persecuted (Stuart and Sundeen, 1995).
Rumination	Persistent thinking about and discussion of a particular subject (Rawlins et al, 1993).

CONTENT REVIEW

I. Paranoid disorders
  A. Definition—concrete, pervasive delusional system, characterized by
      1. Grandiose beliefs
      2. Persecutory beliefs
  B. Psychodynamics
      1. Loss
      2. Emotional pain
      3. Disappointment
      4. Shifts hatred from people who caused the original pain to imaginary oppressors
  C. Common behaviors
      1. Suspicious
      2. Mistrustful ("People are out to get me")
      3. Emotionally distant
      4. Poor insight
      5. Distorts reality
      6. Low self-esteem
      7. Hypervigilance
      8. Difficulty in admitting own error
      9. Takes pride in being correct—superiority

10. Maintains false persecutory beliefs despite evidence or proof
11. Concrete thinking
12. Hypercritical and intolerant of others
13. Hostile
14. Evasive
15. Quarrelsome
16. Aggressive
17. Highly sensitive in perceiving minor injustices, contradictions, and mistakes of others
18. Grandiose delusions
19. Persecutory delusions

D. **Principles underlying paranoid disorders**
   1. Low self-esteem is being defended against
   2. Delusions are an attempt to feel more comfortable with reality
   3. Clients have an extreme need to maintain self-esteem
   4. Delusions serve a purpose in establishing identity and self-esteem
   5. Process of delusion
      a. Denial—"I deny that I dislike myself"
      b. Projection—"It is not that I dislike myself; it is that others dislike me"
      c. Rationalization—"If others dislike me, then they must be out to get me. I am justified in self-defense"
   6. As trust in others increases, need for delusions *decreases*
   7. Behind the anger and suspicion is a lonely, frightened person feeling vulnerable because of low self-esteem

E. **Four types of paranoid disorders**
   1. Paranoid personality
      a. Suspicious
      b. No hallucinations
      c. No delusions
      d. Nonpsychotic
      e. No symptoms of schizophrenia
   2. Paranoid state
      a. Experiences paranoid delusions
      b. No hallucinations
      c. Onset abrupt in response to stress
      d. May be sensitive and suspicious before development of delusions
      e. Prognosis good—subsides when stress decreases
      f. No symptoms of schizophrenia
      g. Psychotic state

3. Paranoia
   a. Single, highly organized delusional system; not bizarre
   b. Client appears normal except for delusional system
   c. No hallucinations
   d. Onset usually in forties
   e. Reserved and sensitive before onset
   f. Poor prognosis once delusional system has set in
   g. No symptoms of schizophrenia
   h. Psychotic state
4. Paranoid schizophrenia
   a. Delusions are bizarre, numerous, changeable
   b. Delusions become less logical as person becomes more disorganized
   c. Experiences hallucinations—persecutory in nature
   d. Gradual onset—late twenties or thirties
   e. Before disorder set in
      (1) Cold
      (2) Withdrawn
      (3) Distrustful
      (4) Resentful
      (5) Argumentative
      (6) Sarcastic
      (7) Defiant
   f. Poor prognosis
   g. All symptoms of schizophrenia present
   h. Psychotic state

II. Application of the nursing process with paranoid disorders

A. **Nursing assessment of client**
   1. Level of trust in others
   2. Level of self-esteem
   3. Suspiciousness
   4. Fears
   5. Feelings of powerlessness
   6. Sleep patterns
   7. Eating patterns
   8. Patterns of interpersonal relationships
   9. Suicidal ideation
   10. Social isolation
   11. Psychomotor disturbances
   12. Presence of hostility

13. Ability to carry out activities of daily living
14. Presence of delusions
15. Presence of hallucinations

B. **Nursing diagnoses**
1. Impaired social interaction
2. Self-esteem disturbance
3. Risk for self-harm
4. Risk for violence
5. Impaired verbal communication
6. Ineffective individual coping
7. Sleep pattern disturbance
8. Social isolation
9. Altered thought process
10. Altered nutrition
11. Noncompliance with treatment
12. Fear
13. Altered sensory perceptions usually visual or auditory

C. **Goals for client**
1. Diminish suspicious behavior
2. Establish trusting relationships with staff
3. Develop sense of reality that is validated by others
4. Express thoughts and feelings verbally and nonaggressively
5. Verbalize increased feelings of self-worth
6. Ingest medication as given
7. Not harm others or self
8. Demonstrate decreased hostility, violence, and aggression
9. Demonstrate decreased delusions, hallucinations, ideas of reference
10. Establish and maintain adequate nutrition, hydration, elimination, and sleep/rest
11. Participate in treatment program

D. **Nursing interventions**
1. Remain calm, nonthreatening, and nonjudgmental
2. Assign the same staff member to consistently work with the client, if possible
3. Respond honestly to client at all times
4. Follow through on commitments made to client
5. Tell the client that you do not share his/her interpretations of an event, while acknowledging the feelings involved
6. Provide a daily schedule of activities
7. Help client identify adaptive diversionary activities, such as recreation and groups

8. Gradually introduce client to group situations
9. Use role playing to help identify feelings and thoughts
10. Give positive reinforcement for successes
11. Refocus conversation to reality-based topics
12. Do not argue with delusions; simply point out that you do not share the same beliefs
13. Use concrete, specific words
14. Identify feelings presented by client during interactions
15. Give clear information related to confidentiality issues
16. Focus on reality-based ideas
17. Inform client how he/she is perceived by others, such as suspicious or intimidating
18. Do not be secretive with client
19. Convey to client that he/she will be safe
20. Do not whisper in client's presence
21. Do not allow client to ruminate
22. Observe client closely for agitation; decrease stimuli as appropriate
23. Involve in noncompetitive tasks
24. Provide opportunity to complete small tasks and give support for success
25. Observe eating, drinking, and elimination patterns
26. Observe sleeping pattern
27. Limit physical contact
28. Do not mix medications with food

E. **Evaluation**
1. Suspicious behavior has decreased to a manageable level
2. Client trusts staff enough to nonaggressively verbalize needs, feelings, and thoughts
3. Client verbalizes increased sense of worth
4. Client is able to participate in small-group activities
5. Adequate nutrition, hydration, elimination, and sleep patterns have been established
6. Delusions and hallucinations are absent or do not interrupt activities of daily living
7. Client is compliant with treatment plan
8. Client is not harmful to self or others

REVIEW QUESTIONS

1. A client refuses to eat food sent up on individual trays from the hospital kitchen. The client shouts,"You want to kill me." The client has lost 8 pounds in 4 days. In discussion of this problem with the assigned staff member, which statement by the nurse indicates an accurate interpretation of this client's needs?
   a. "The client is malnourished and may require tube feedings"
   b. "The client is terrified. Ask the kitchen to send foods that are not easily contaminated such as baked potatoes."
   c. "Continue to observe the client. When the client gets hungry enough, the client will eat."
   d. "The client appears frightened. Spend more time with the client, showing a warm affection."

2. For clients with paranoid disorders, which would be an initial goal?
   a. The clients will diminish suspicious behavior
   b. The clients will express thoughts and feelings verbally
   c. The clients will develop a sense of trust of reality that is validated by others
   d. The clients will establish trusting relationships with staff

3. The student nurse is discussing paranoid disorders at lunch with the nurse manager. Which statement by the student indicates correct knowledge about this disorder?
   a. Clients have a minimal need to maintain self-esteem
   b. As trust in others increases, the need for delusions decreases
   c. Hallucinations make clients in the paranoid state feel more comfortable with reality
   d. These clients are lonely and frightened without an ability to exhibit anger or hostility

4. A client diagnosed with paranoia has discussed 10 times in the last 3 hours the issue of breakfast with the psychiatric assistant. The nurse would document this behavior as
   a. Hypervigilance
   b. Repetitive delusion
   c. Parroting
   d. Rumination

5. The least severe type of paranoid disorder is
   a. Paranoid schizophrenia
   b. Paranoid personality
   c. Paranoia
   d. Paranoid state

ANSWERS, RATIONALES, AND TEST-TAKING TIPS

Rationales	Test-Taking Tips

1. Correct answer: b

Currently this client is displaying paranoid behavior. The client is verbalizing fearful thoughts, so during this time foods should be given that are wrapped or sealed to encourage the client to eat. The actions of the nurse should be directed at diminishing the suspicious behavior, establishing a trusting relationship, and assisting the client to develop a sense of reality.

Note that all of the initial statements are correct for this situation. However, in option *a* the tube feedings are premature at this time; in option *c* the statement is incorrect; and in option *d* the intervention is inappropriate when the client is exhibiting paranoid behaviors.

2. Correct answer: a

The other goals would be incorporated but not in the initial stages of care.

The key words in the stem are "the initial goal." Note that in this type of question all of the responses will be correct. Your task is to prioritize the options.

3. Correct answer: b

In paranoid disorders low self-esteem is being defended against. It is delusions that make clients in the paranoid state feel more comfortable with reality. Behind the anger and suspicion is a lonely, frightened person feeling vulnerable because of low self-esteem.

Reading carefully and slowly to identify the key words, "indicates correct knowledge" will lead to the correct answer selection. Use your "go with what you know" approach to eliminate options *a, c,* and *d*. Logical thinking tells you that as trust increases the clinical findings would more than likely decrease.

4. **Correct answer: d**

Rumination is the persistent thinking about and discussion of a particular subject. Hypervigilance is a persistent sense of danger which involves physiological arousal and heightened attention to the environment while in search of early warning signs of impending danger. A repetitive delusion is a false belief that keeps occurring. Parroting is the repeating of the statement of another.

The approach for this question is to eliminate the incorrect options. Think logically. In option *a* vigilance is looking for, so eliminate it as an answer. In option *b* delusions are false belief and the stem gives no information to support this as a selection. In option *c* think of a parrot that will repeat what a person says. The stem gives no information about repeating words or phrases.

5. **Correct answer: b**

The paranoid disorders from least to greatest severity are: paranoid personality, paranoid state, paranoia, and paranoid schizophrenia.

Think logically and use common sense. A personality would precede a paranoid state. The most severe condition would be the schizophrenia. This leaves the paranoia to be one step below the most severe.

Disorders of Childhood and Adolescence

STUDY OUTCOMES

After completing this chapter, the reader will be able to do the following:

▼ Describe common medical diagnoses used for children with emotional disorders.

▼ Discuss the major categories of data included in the assessment of a child's health status.

▼ Describe nursing interventions to be included in the plan of care for children.

▼ Identify the major categories of data to be collected in the assessment of an adolescent's health status.

▼ Discuss common areas of conflict during adolescence.

▼ Describe specific problems often experienced by adolescents.

▼ Apply the nursing process when working with children and adolescents.

▼ Discuss the various disorders common in adolescence.

KEY TERMS

Coprolalia	Use of socially unacceptable words, frequently obscene.
Echolalia	Involuntary, parrotlike repetition of words spoken by others.
Encopresis	Repeated passage of feces into places not appropriate, whether voluntary or involuntary, by a child at least 4 years old, often caused by constipation and watery colonic contents bypassing fecal masses (Stuart and Sundeen, 1995).
Enuresis	Repeated voiding of urine during the day or night into bed or clothes, whether voluntary or involuntary, by a child at least 5 years old (Stuart and Sundeen, 1995).
Metaphorical language	Language only understood by those familiar with the person's communication style.
Pervasive development disorders	Severe impairment in social skills or communication skills, or the presence of stereotyped behavior, interests, and activities.
Pica	Eating nonnutritive substances.
Primary process thinking	Primitive thought process normally kept unconscious by use of repression; it is autistic in nature.
Tic	Sudden, rapid, recurrent, stereotyped motor movement or vocalization.

CONTENT REVIEW

I. Psychodynamics of childhood disorders
A. Poorly functioning ego
1. Cannot tolerate frustration
2. Needs immediate gratification
3. When frustrated, behavior becomes
   a. Panic
   b. Aggressive
   c. Destructive
4. Excitement of the forbidden
   a. Longs to do forbidden things
   b. Often excitation spreads to a group of children
5. New situations are frightening and overstimulating
6. Insensitive to feelings of others

      7. Difficulty in functioning by social rules
      8. Ignores rules
      9. Does not learn from mistakes
    10. Cannot see own role in problems
    11. Resists forming relationships with healthy adults
        a. Mistrust
        b. Fear of rejection
    12. Impaired object relations
    13. Narcissistic
    14. Primary process thinking

B. Family psychodynamics

    1. Child is the symptom bearer for the family
    2. Special meaning for parents at child's birth
        a. Only child
        b. Chronic illness
    3. Parents have been inadequately parented themselves
    4. Blurring of ego boundaries
        a. Roles overlap or are reversed
        b. Child parents the parents
        c. Feelings may be projected between family members
        d. High levels of anxiety travel from one family member to another
        e. Poor differentiation of family members

II. Types of childhood disorders

A. Pervasive developmental disorders

    1. Childhood psychosis
    2. Dysfunctional in social relationships
    3. High anxiety levels
    4. Self-mutilation
    5. High impairment
    6. Poor prognosis
    7. Autistic disorder
        a. Impaired social interaction
            (1) Failure to develop peer relationships
            (2) Little or no interest in friendships
            (3) Lack of seeking to share enjoyment with others
            (4) Engages in solitary activities
        b. Impaired communication
            (1) Delay in or lack of language
            (2) Difficulty conversing with others
            (3) Lack of make-believe play

         (4)   Tone of voice may be abnormal

         (5)   Repetitive words

         (6)   Metaphorical language

         (7)   Inability to understand questions

  c. Restricted activity and interests

         (1)   Preoccupied with narrow interest, such as football statistics

         (2)   Resists trivial changes, such as new curtains

         (3)   Insists on following routines, such as following same route to school every day

         (4)   Stereotyped body movements, such as rocking, clapping, finger flicking

         (5)   Abnormal posture, such as walking on tiptoe

         (6)   Preoccupied with parts of objects, such as buttons or parts of body

         (7)   Fascinated with movement, such as spinning wheels of toys

  d. 75% function at retarded level (IQ 35 to 50)

  e. Behavioral symptoms

         (1)   Hyperactivity

         (2)   Short attention span

         (3)   Impulsivity

         (4)   Self-injurious behaviors (head banging)

         (5)   Temper tantrums

         (6)   Oversensitivity to sounds or touch

         (7)   Abnormalities in eating (pica)

         (8)   Mood abnormalities (giggling, weeping)

  f. Incidence

         (1)   2 to 5 cases per 10,000 individuals

         (2)   Onset before age 3

         (3)   In one third of cases partial independence is possible

         (4)   Usually continue to exhibit problems in social interaction and communication

    (Modified from American Psychiatric Association, 1994)

8. Childhood disintegrative disorder

  a. Regression in functioning after a period of normal development

         (1)   Communication

         (2)   Social relationships

         (3)   Play

  b. Loss of

        (1) Expressive or receptive language
        (2) Social skills
        (3) Bowel or bladder control
        (4) Play
        (5) Motor skills

   c. Usually associated with mental retardation
   d. EEG abnormalities
   e. Seizure disorder
   f. Incidence
        (1) Very rare
        (2) More common among males
        (3) Onset before age 10
        (4) Duration is usually lifelong
           (a) Social difficulties
           (b) Communication difficulties
           (c) Behavioral difficulties
     (Modified from American Psychiatric Association, 1994)

B. Attention deficit-hyperactivity disorder

  1. Persistent pattern of inattention and/or hyperactivity—impulsivity
   a. Academic
   b. Occupational
   c. Social situations
  2. Does not follow through on requests or fails to complete schoolwork, chores, small tasks
  3. Difficulty organizing tasks
  4. Impatience
  5. Difficulty waiting one's turn
  6. Failure to wait for directions
  7. Low frustration tolerance
  8. Rejection by peers
  9. Poor self-esteem
  10. Incidence
   a. 3% to 5% of school-age children
   b. Disorder is stable through adolescence
   c. In most individuals behaviors stop in adolescence and adulthood
   d. Some adults retain some behaviors
   (Modified from American Psychiatric Association, 1994)

C. Conduct disorder

  1. Repetitive and persistent pattern of behavior in which the rights of others and/or societal norms are violated

2. Occurs up to age 18 or over 18 if criteria for antisocial personality disorder are not met
3. Characteristics
    a. Aggression toward people and animals
        (1) Bullies
        (2) Physically cruel
        (3) Forced sexual activity
        (4) Theft
    b. Destruction of property
        (1) Setting fires
        (2) Destroying property, such as breaking windows
    c. Deceitfulness or theft
        (1) Shoplifting
        (2) Forgery
        (3) Lying for self-gain
        (4) Breaking into house, car
    d. Violation of rules
        (1) Runaway behavior
        (2) Truancy
        (3) Stays out at night despite parental rules
4. Incidence
    a. Males under 18—6% to 16% of population
    b. Females under 18—2% to 9% of population
    c. Usually begins in late childhood or early adolescence
    d. Onset rare after 16 years of age
    e. In majority of clients remission occurs by adulthood
    f. In adulthood may appear as antisocial personality disorder
    g. Early onset predicts worse prognosis
    h. These clients are also at risk as adults for mood or anxiety disorders, somatoform disorders, and substance-related disorders
    (Modified from American Psychiatric Association, 1994)
D. **Oppositional defiant disorder**
    1. Negativistic, hostile behavior toward authority figures
    2. Argues with adults
    3. Defies rules of adults
    4. Deliberately annoys people
    5. Blames others for own mistakes
    6. Vindictive
    7. Tests of limits
    8. Behaviors present at home and sometimes at school

9. Incidence
   a. 2% to 16% of population
   b. Usually evident before 8 years of age
   c. Often leads to conduct disorder
   (Modified from American Psychiatric Association, 1994)
E. **Pica eating disorder**
   1. Persistent eating of nonnutritive substances
   2. Younger children
      a. Paint
      b. Plaster
      c. String
      d. Hair
      e. Cloth
   3. Older children
      a. Animal droppings
      b. Sand
      c. Insects
      d. Leaves
      e. Pebbles
   4. Usually lasts several months
   5. Occasionally lasts to adolescence
   6. Onset usually occurs in infancy
F. **Tourette's disorder**
   1. Multiple motor tics—head, torso, upper and lower limbs
   2. Vocal tics—clicks, grunts, barks, sniffs, snorts, coughs, swears
   3. Complex motor tics—deep knee bends/twirling
   4. Causes significant impairment in functioning
   5. Obsessions
   6. Compulsions
   7. Age of onset—2 to 18 years
   8. Symptoms may decrease during adolescence
   9. Symptoms may disappear by adulthood
   10. Genetic vulnerability to disorder
   11. Incidence
       a. Occurs in 4 to 5 individuals per 10,000
       b. May occur as early as 2 years but must be before 18
       c. Duration is usually for life, with periods of remission from weeks to years
       d. Usually behaviors diminish during adolescence and adulthood
       (Modified from American Psychiatric Association, 1994)

G. Encopresis disorder
  1. Constipation and fecal retention
  2. Watery colonic contents bypass hard fecal masses and pass through rectum
  3. Confused with diarrhea
  4. May be involuntary or intentional
  5. May cause embarrassment
  6. Results in social ostracism
  7. Decreased self-esteem
  8. Anger, punishment by care providers
  9. Incidence
    a. 1% of 5-year-olds
    b. More common in males
    c. May persist with intermittent exacerbations but rarely is chronic
  (Modified from American Psychiatric Association, 1994)
H. Enuresis disorder
  1. Repeated voiding of urine during day (diurnal) or at night (nocturnal) into bed or clothes
  2. May be involuntary or intentional
  3. Impairment in social and academic functioning
  4. Results in social ostracism
  5. Decreased self-esteem
  6. Anger, punishment by care providers
  7. Predisposing factors
    a. Lax toilet training
    b. Psychosocial stress
    c. Low bladder volume threshold for involuntary voiding
    d. Excessive water drinking
    e. Spinal cord injury
    f. Medical diseases
      (1) Diabetes mellitus
      (2) Diabetes insipidus
      (3) Epilepsy
      (4) Cystitis
  8. Incidence
    a. At age 5
      (1) 7% of males
      (2) 3% of females
    b. At age 10
      (1) 3% of males
      (2) 2% of females

    c. At age 18
       (1) 1% of males
       (2) Less than 1% of females
    (Modified from American Psychiatric Association, 1994)

I. Separation anxiety disorder
1. Excessive anxiety related to separation from home or from significant others
2. When separated needs to stay in touch (phone calls)
3. Extreme homesickness
4. Preoccupied with fears of accidents or illnesses to significant others
5. Difficulty at bedtime
6. Nightmares
7. Physical complaints
    a. Stomachaches
    b. Headaches
    c. Nausea
    d. Vomiting
8. Depression
9. Refusal to go to school or elsewhere
10. Incidence
    a. Occurs in 4% of children and adolescents
    b. Periods of exacerbation and remission
    c. May persist for many years
    (Modified from American Psychiatric Association, 1994)

J. Reactive attachment disorder
1. Disturbance in social relatedness
2. Inhibited type
    a. Failure to initiate social interactions
    b. Failure to respond to social interactions
3. Disinhibited type
    a. Lack of selectivity in choice of attachments
    b. Attachments with strangers
4. Causes
    a. Disregard of child's basic needs
    b. Physical abuse
    c. Repeated changes in primary care provider
5. Incidence
    a. Very uncommon
    b. Occurs before age 5
    c. Considerable improvement or remission may occur if supportive environment is provided
    (Modified from American Psychiatric Association, 1994)

III. Application of the nursing process with childhood disorders

A. Nursing assessment
1. Use play materials to decrease child's anxiety during assessment process
2. Appearance
   a. Physical size
   b. Dress
   c. Hygiene
   d. Posture
   e. Handicaps
3. Defense mechanisms—defenses the child uses to cope with anxiety
4. Neuromusculature
   a. Motor movements
   b. Coordinated movements
5. Thought process
   a. Logical
   b. Cohesive
   c. Flight of ideas
   d. Loose associations
   e. Hallucinations
   f. Delusions
6. Fantasy
   a. Ability to fantasize
   b. Wish fulfillment
   c. Dreams
7. Concept of self
   a. Self-esteem
   b. Self-image
   c. Self-ideal
8. Orientation
   a. Concept of time
   b. Ability to perceive who and where he or she is
9. Superego
   a. Value system
   b. Right from wrong
   c. Response to limit setting
10. Estimated intelligence quotient (IQ)
    a. General information
    b. Age-appropriate tasks
11. Interpersonal relationships

        a. How the child relates to peers
        b. Peers close in age?
        c. Best friend?
        d. Ability to relate to adults
        e. Does child see adults as hostile enemies?

12. Activities
        a. Type
        b. Energy level
        c. Ability to engage in solitary and group activities

13. History of symptoms
        a. Precipitating problem
        b. Growth and development
        c. Family life
        d. School adjustment
        e. Medical status

(Modified from Stuart and Sundeen, 1995)

B. Nursing diagnoses
1. Impaired verbal communication
2. Ineffective family coping
3. Ineffective individual coping
4. Altered family processes
5. Fear
6. Altered growth and development
7. Bowel incontinence
8. Risk for injury
9. Altered nutrition
10. Anxiety
11. Impaired physical mobility
12. Altered sensory perceptions
13. Impaired social interaction
14. Self-esteem disturbance
15. Altered thought process
16. Risk for violence

C. Goals for client
1. Client will exhibit decreased anxiety
2. Client will exhibit positive interpersonal relationships
3. Client will exhibit increased self-esteem
4. Client will exhibit effective communication
5. Client will exhibit freedom from injury
6. Client will exhibit improved physical health
7. Client will exhibit contact with reality
8. Client will exhibit adaptive coping behaviors

D. **Nursing interventions**
1. Family therapy
   a. Educate parents about role in problem
   b. Encourage parents to take responsibility for change
   c. Child is not the problem but a manifestation of problem in family
2. Group therapy
   a. Activity
   b. Reality testing
   c. Impulse control
   d. Self-esteem
   e. Social skills
3. Individual therapy—play therapy
   a. Work through conflicts
   b. Master developmental tasks
   c. Tool for communication
   d. Master past experiences
4. Milieu therapy—explore daily life events
5. Psychopharmacology (Table 16-1)
6. Supportive ego intervention
   a. Exert external control
   b. Maintain ego function
   c. Show empathy for frustration
   d. Stay with child during loss of control
   e. Keep child engaged
   f. Enforce rules and regulations
7. Interpretive ego function
   a. Gain insight
   b. Make changes
8. Behavior modification
   a. Child rewarded with points or tokens
   b. Maladaptive behavior ignored or punished with timeout
   c. Timeout—brief period away from group
   d. Goal: to internalize child's self-control
E. **Evaluation**
1. Has brief but common hospitalizations
2. Able to relate to peers, adults, parents
3. Able to care for self and possessions
4. Responds to limits, rules, and routines
5. Has insight into problems
6. Willing to change
7. Able to use program activities in recreation and learning
8. Feels good about self as a person

Table 16-1. **Child Psychiatric Disorders and Drug Treatments**

Disorder	Drug Class	Comments/Nursing Considerations
Attention deficit-hyperactivity disorder (ADHD)	Stimulants—Benzedrine, Ritalin, Cylert	Used when primary symptoms are manifest in school
		Less reliable in preschooler and adolescent
	Antidepressants—imipramine (Tofranil) most common	Once-a-day dose and improved monitoring of compliance and toxicity using plasma levels
		Monitor cardiac status and signs of overdose
	Antipsychotics—haloperidol (Haldol)	Sometimes used in combination with stimulants for symptomatic relief
Conduct disorders	Antipsychotics, stimulants—Benzedrine, Ritalin, Cyclert	May improve a child's capacity to benefit from social and educational interventions
Enuresis	Antidepressants—imipramine (Tofranil)	Used when an immediate therapeutic effect is necessary due to severe emotional distress
Eating disorders	Antihistamines—cyproheptadine, antipsychotics	Anorexia nervosa
	Antidepressants—imipramine (Tofranil)	Bulimia
Affective disorders: depression	Antidepressants—imipramine (Tofranil)	Careful diagnosis is necessary to differentiate depression from normal feeling states
Tic disorders: Tourette's disorder	Antipsychotics—haloperidol Alpha-adrenergic agonist—clonidine	Stimulants are avoided because they worsen symptoms
Pervasive developmental disorders	Antipsychotics—Haldol	Used to treat agitation, insomnia, stereotypic movements

Continued.

Table 16-1. Child Psychiatric Disorders and Drug Treatments—cont'd

Disorder	Drug Class	Comments/Nursing Considerations
Mental retardation with psychiatric symptoms and behavioral problems	Antipsychotics—Haldol	Used to control behavior and psychiatric complaints
	Antidepressants— imipramine (Tofranil)	Treat affective symptoms
	Stimulants— Benzedrine, Ritalin, Cylert	Treat AD-HD
	Lithium	Helps control aggression
Separation anxiety disorder	Antidepressants— imipramine (Tofranil)	Effective at high doses Speculative: panic disorder symptoms
Schizophrenic disorder	Antipsychotics—Haldol	As with adults, choice of drug depends on prior efficacy and the spectrum of pharmacological properties
Anxiety, impulse problems, transient insomnia, acute EPS	Antihistamines— Benadryl	Tolerance to sedative effects may develop

Modified from Stuart G and Sundeen S, *Principles and practice of psychiatric nursing,* ed 5, St Louis, 1995, Mosby.

IV. Adolescence

    A. Issues confronting adolescence

        1. Body image

           a. Compares self to peers

           b. The greater the divergence from the rest of the group, the greater the anxiety

           c. Extreme concern with body changes can lead to hypochondriasis

        2. Identity

           a. Second individuation process

           b. Tests self by going to extremes

           c. Rebelliousness and negativism show movement to autonomy

      d. Feelings of isolation, loneliness, confusion

      e. Mourns loss of childhood

      f. Needs support or depression may result

      g. Family members need clear boundaries

3. Independence

      a. Unconscious longing to be dependent

      b. Sees independence as freedom from parental control

      c. "If one acts adult, one is adult" (Stuart and Sundeen, 1995)

      d. Exposes himself/herself to situations he/she cannot handle

      e. Regresses back to childlike behavior

      f. Projects ambivalence about independence onto parents

      g. Blames parents for treating him/her like a child

4. Sexuality

      a. Sexual feelings intensify

      b. Fusion of sexual impulses with love

      c. Rejection of love for parents related to incestuous and homosexual connections in thought process

5. Social role

      a. Responds intensely to persons

      b. Hero worship

      c. Crushes

      d. Poor discrimination in attachments

      e. Chum relationships help solidify identity

      f. Peer group important

6. Sexual behavior

      a. Uses fantasy

      b. May feel guilt and shame about feelings

      c. Masturbation common

      d. Mutual masturbation used for tension release

      (Modified from Stuart and Sundeen, 1995)

B. **Behavioral disorders of adolescence**

1. Dysfunctional sexuality

      a. Victims of sexual abuse as children

      b. Early sexual experimentation—peer pressure

      c. Unprotected sexual intercourse

         (1) Increased risk of pregnancy

         (2) Increased risk for acquired immunodeficiency syndrome (AIDS) and sexually transmitted diseases

    d. Sexual promiscuity
       (1) Underlying depression and anxiety
       (2) Reinforces poor self-concept
       (3) Prostitution, both boys and girls
    e. Experimental homosexual activity
       (1) Usually evolves into heterosexual orientation
       (2) May create anxiety about heterosexuality
       (3) High incidence of suicidality
    f. Sexual aggression
       (1) Frustration
       (2) Anger
       (3) Deprivation
       (4) Rape victimizer
    g. Unwed motherhood
       (1) Escape from family situation
       (2) Defense against homosexual feelings
       (3) Validation of bad role in family

2. Adolescent suicide
    a. Response after loss of a meaningful relationship
    b. Healthcare providers should take suicide attempts seriously
    c. Second cause of death in adolescents
    d. 17% increase in adolescent suicides since 1950
    e. Tend to be impulsive
    f. History of unsuccessful attempts to solve problems
    g. Feeling isolated and lonely
    h. Feeling powerless
    i. Academic problems
    j. Unrealistic parental expectations
    k. History of child abuse
    l. Unstable or chaotic home life
    m. High number of school changes
    n. Attempted or completed suicide by close friend
    o. Questioning sexual orientation
    p. Dynamics
       (1) Feels rejected and unwanted by family
       (2) Unfulfilled need for love
       (3) Overwhelming sense of loss

3. Runaway behavior
    a. Unconscious conflicts
    b. Parental rejection

     c. Inconsistent parenting

     d. Dependence-independence conflict

     e. Runs away to prove autonomy

     f. Desires to earn money for substances

4. Conduct disorders (see childhood section)

5. Violence (Clinical Example 16-1)

     a. Has violent role models

     b. Does not learn healthy expression of aggression

     c. Fears loss of control over destructive impulses

     d. Needs to recognize fears and be reassured of external limits. Example: "We will help you to maintain control."

6. Substance use disorder—to relieve tension

     a. 50% to 95% of adolescents have used drugs at least once

     b. Casual users

       (1) Alcohol

       (2) Marijuana

       (3) Peer pressure

Clinical Example 16-1. Adolescent Violence

Client was a 14-year-old boy referred for treatment for violent outbursts at home. When frustrated he would break and destroy objects in his path. He was an only child, adopted shortly after birth by a couple in their forties who were unable to have children. Now his parents, who were about 55 years of age, were increasingly frightened by his aggressive outbursts. They had also felt powerless with his childhood temper tantrums and had consistently responded to outbursts by attempting to limit frustrating situations. They felt guilty and inadequate about his being an adopted child and continually made attempts to reassure him of their love for him. They consequently reinforced his lack of control by assuming these outbursts were results of his fear of being unloved, and would offer peace offerings of gifts and rewards. The client assumed he was omnipotent, successfully controlling his parents, but was fearful that he could not control his anger. Acknowledging his fear of loss of control, applying external controls, and pointing out areas of his ability for responsibility and control resulted in a gradual decrease in outbursts. First the outbursts became more limited as the client began breaking specific things that he did not value. Then he progressed to an elimination of violent outbursts.

Modified from Stuart G and Sundeen S, *Principles and practice of psychiatric nursing,* ed 5, St Louis, 1995, Mosby.

      c. Sociological users
         (1) Social process
         (2) Form groups free of social convention
         (3) Relief from boredom
         (4) Mystical revelation
      d. Sick users
         (1) Mask or correct problems
         (2) Serious interpersonal difficulties
         (3) Prefer drugs to people
         (4) Critical of society
         (Modified from Stuart and Sundeen, 1995)

7. Hypochondriasis
    a. Intense anxiety about health
    b. General feelings of inadequacy
    c. Responds to changes in body with increased intensity

8. Weight problems
    a. Eating disorders common
    b. Emphasis on thinness
    c. Self-control and social success are culturally rewarded
    d. Underlying conflict is sexual
        (1) Thinness or heaviness—denying sexuality
        (2) Excessive eating—symbolic of taking in love

9. School phobia
    a. Neurotic anxiety
    b. Fears related to independence and maturation
    c. School becomes focus of fears

10. Occult involvement
    a. Alienated from family
    b. Socially isolated
    c. Attracted to bizarre
    d. Negative
    e. Fatalistic
    f. Relies on superstition to deal with powerlessness
    g. Beliefs give sense of control
    h. Satanism
        (1) Common in boys
        (2) Symbolizes evil
    i. Witchcraft
        (1) Common in girls
        (2) Manipulating spirits
    j. Behaviors
        (1) Sleep disturbances

            (2)   Suicidal ideation

            (3)   Substance abuse

            (4)   Fantasy role play (Dungeons and Dragons)

            (5)   Rituals

            (6)   Preference for heavy metal music

C. Application of the nursing process with the adolescent

  1. Nursing assessment

    a. Growth and development

    b. Biophysical status (illness, accidents)

    c. Emotional status (relationships, affect, mental status, suicidal or homicidal ideation)

    d. Cultural, religious, and socioeconomic background

    e. Performance of activities of daily living at home and school

    f. Coping patterns

    g. Interaction patterns with family and peers

    h. Perception of health

    i. Availability of resources

  2. Nursing diagnoses

    a. Anxiety

    b. Body image disturbance

    c. Ineffective family coping

    d. Ineffective individual coping

    e. Fear

    f. Altered growth and development

    g. Hopelessness

    h. Risk for injury

    i. Altered nutrition

    j. Personal identity disturbance

    k. Powerlessness

    l. Self-esteem disturbance

    m. Sexual dysfunction

    n. Sleep pattern disturbance

    o. Risk for violence

  3. Goals for client

    a. Client will have adequate impulse control

    b. Client will interact with other clients

    c. Client will decrease rebelliousness

    d. Client will not harm self or others

    e. Client will accept limit setting

    f. Client will express sexuality appropriately

    g. Client will have increased self-esteem

      h. Client will have decreased anxiety related to independent actions

      i. Client will talk about feelings with staff

      j. Client will incorporate a value system

      k. Client will manage aggression effectively

4. Nursing interventions

    a. Family therapy

    b. Group therapy

      (1) Peer support

      (2) Peer feedback

      (3) Interpersonal skill learning

      (4) Ego identity formation through peer contact

      (5) Male and female cotherapists

      (6) Work out family conflicts

    c. Therapeutic alliance

      (1) Nurse aligns with healthy part of ego

      (2) Critical understanding of inner experience

      (3) Interpretation of feeling states

      (4) Link between feelings and behavior

      (5) Point out behavior is motivated by feelings

      (6) Neutral attitude toward all behavior

      (7) Point out self-critical tendencies

      (8) Point out seeing things in extremes

      (9) Distinguish between thoughts and actions ("anger isn't killing")

      (10) Encourage expression of emotion

      (11) Continue meeting despite provocative behavior

    d. Silence

      (1) Frightening to adolescents

      (2) Brief silences are tolerable

    e. Confidentiality

      (1) Do not make promises not to tell parents

      (2) Dangerous thoughts or actions must be shared

      (3) You will tell them when you will be disclosing information

    f. Ignore negative comments about not needing treatment—remain neutral

    g. Admit having a lack of knowledge in areas such as this; provides role modeling against the need to be perfect

    h. Set only essential limits that may be enforced

    i. Have client utilize art, music, journaling for expressing feelings

     j. Explore with clients the consequences of their actions
     k. Encourage participation in unit activities
     l. Point out strengths
     m. Give positive feedback on efforts toward independence
     n. Open communication between client and parent
     o. Set up graduated, clearly specified responsibilities
     p. Help client choose issues of disagreement with parents and negotiate change
     q. Ignore sexually provocative behavior when used to gain attention

5. Evaluation
     a. Is comfortable with beginning independence from parents
     b. Is comfortable with self and body image
     c. Verbalizes feelings appropriately without harm to self or others
     d. Follows rules and regulations
     e. Has established short-term goals

REVIEW QUESTIONS

1. Parents are at the clinic with a child diagnosed with attention deficit-hyperactivity disorder. Which group of characteristics would the nurse most likely observe in the waiting room of the clinic? The child
    a. Plays with two children in the waiting room
    b. Runs over and turns on the video player without listening to the parents' directions
    c. Constantly wiggles a leg when waiting to take a turn at the board game
    d. Puts the toy truck back into the playbox only after visiting with three other children and their parents

2. During the assessment of a very young client's affective responses to sexual abuse by a parent, the nurse would most likely identify that the client
    a. Feels responsible and guilty for not stopping the abuse
    b. Feels that the other parent will not blame but rather support the client
    c. Exhibits the defense mechanism of bargaining to manage the trauma
    d. Isolates the emotions from the experience by performing rituals for anxiety reduction

3. A pregnant 12-year-old comments, "It will be so much fun to have a little baby around the house. I know I can love the baby and the baby will love me." What is the best reply by the nurse?
    a. "I'm happy to see that you are looking forward and are happy about this baby"
    b. "Tell me about your parents' reaction to your pregnancy"
    c. "Let's talk about how you think that your life will be different after the baby is born"
    d. "Babies are a lot of work, as well as fun. What changes have you made in your room for the baby?"

4. Which classification of drugs may be used with children to treat enuresis?
    a. Tricyclic antidepressants
    b. Major tranquilizers
    c. Antianxiety agents
    d. Hypnotic

ANSWERS, RATIONALES, AND TEST-TAKING TIPS

Rationales	Test-Taking Tips

1. **Correct answer: b**

   The failure to wait for directions is typical of the attention deficit-hyperactivity disorder (AD-HD). The other behaviors are typical of children. In option *b* the child waits for a turn. In option *d* the child gets distracted to visit with others; however, the child does complete the task. In AD-HD children have difficulty completing homework, chores or small tasks.

   Make this question simple by approaching it logically. Option *a* is normal for a child to play with 2 children. In option *c* the child exhibits an ability to wait. In option *d* the child completes the small task of returning the toy to the box. These can be clustered. Only in option *b* does the child's behavior exhibit a variation from the other options. Select option *b*.

2. **Correct answer: d**

   The very young child is more likely to preform rituals to deal with the situation. The other options are too high of a level of behavior for a young child.

   The important words to note in this question are "very young child." Read the option with this in mind to eliminate options *a, b,* and *c* since they are more behavior of older children.

3. **Correct answer: c**

   This reply, an open ended response, will help the preteen to more realistically prepare for the infant. Option *a* is nontherapeutic since it is giving approval. Option *b* is incorrect since it focuses on the parents instead of the client. Option *d* is a change of the subject and incorrect.

   The best reply by the nurse is to get the preteen to talk about how she expects things to be after the baby is born. The need is to have her discuss the situation in more specific terms.

4. **Correct answer: a**

The tricyclic antidepressant imipramine hydrochloride (Tofranil) has been indicated for the treatment of enuresis in children over the age of 6. It has an antineuritic effect due to anticholinergic actions. The other drugs have no effect for children with enuresis.

Recall tip: The *tricyclic*, *T*rofranil, is used in *t*ots for enuresis ("*t-t*" at night—"t-t" is an expression of urinating similar to pee-pee that is commonly used by little children/tots).

Disorders of the Older Adult

STUDY OUTCOMES

After completing this chapter, the reader will be able to do the following:

▼ Describe psychiatric disorders associated with aging.

▼ Discuss the major biological and psychosocial theories of aging.

▼ Describe losses common in the older adult population.

▼ Discuss bereavement, suicide, isolation, and loneliness as issues of aging.

▼ Apply the nursing process with the older adult experiencing mental disorders.

KEY TERMS

Remote memory	Recall of events that occurred in the distant past.
Reunion fantasies	Wishes to join a deceased loved one in the afterlife.
Short-term memory	Recall of recent events.
Sundown syndrome	Disorientation, confusion, and apathy in the late afternoon and evening.
Sunrise syndrome	Early morning confusion.

CONTENT REVIEW

I. Theories of aging
  A. **Biological**
    1. Wear-and-tear theory—structural and functional changes may be accelerated by abuse and decelerated by care
    2. Stress-adaptation theory
      a. Positive and negative effects of stress on physiological and psychological development
      b. Stress accelerates the aging process
  B. **Psychosocial theories**
    1. Disengagement theory (University of Chicago Committee on Human Development)
      a. Older adults and society mutually withdraw
      b. Older people enjoy the company of people their own age
    2. Activity theory (M.F. Lowenthal)
      a. Activity is most positive environment for the older adult
      b. Should remain active as long as possible
    3. Life review (Robert Butler)
      a. Return to consciousness of past experiences
      b. Resurgence of unresolved conflicts
      c. Reintegration of experiences
      d. Meaning to life
      e. Preparation for death
      f. Decreased anxiety and fear
      g. Righting of earlier wrongs

II. Issues of aging
  A. **Memory loss**
    1. Loss of short-term memory
    2. Access to memory slows with age

3. Causes
   a. Stress
   b. Crisis
   c. Depression
   d. Sense of worthlessness
B. Withdrawal
   1. Fear of losses
   2. Prolonged grief
   3. Organic intellectual impairment
C. Confusion
   1. Inattention
   2. Memory deficits
   3. Inappropriate verbalizations
   4. Disruptive behavior
   5. Noncompliance
   6. Problems performing activities of daily living
   7. Sunrise syndrome
      a. Hangover effects of nighttime medications
      b. Insomnia
   8. Sundown syndrome
   9. Drug overdose due to malabsorption of medications
D. Paranoia
   1. Reaction to loss, loneliness
   2. Perceive threat to family, friends, neighbors
   3. May be precipitated by relocation to new environment
   4. Aloof
   5. Fearful
   6. Oversensitive
   7. Secretive
   8. High risk for victimization by others
E. Dysfunctional grieving
   1. Definition—a prolonged grief over a real or imagined loss
   2. Is influenced by attitude toward own aging and death
   3. Symptoms
      a. Weight loss
      b. Anorexia
      c. Fatigue
      d. Apathy
      e. Loss of interest
      f. Psychomotor retardation
      g. Loss of hope

F. Suicide
 1. 25% of suicides are older adults
 2. Higher risk—isolated older adult
 3. May result from lost family or friends
 4. May result from changes in body function
 5. Types of suicidal behaviors
    a. Risk-taking
    b. Refusal to eat
    c. Misuse of substances
    d. Noncompliance with medical regimen
G. Hypochondriasis
 1. Definition—preoccupation with physical and emotional health
 2. Concerns expressed through body complaints
 3. Complaints reflect an expression of underlying needs and fears
 4. Nursing intervention—take all complaints seriously
H. Insomnia
 1. Interrupted sleep
 2. Morning exhaustion
 3. Daytime napping
 4. Less sleep is required with age
 5. Lack of exercise, limited mobility, side effects of drugs
    contribute to insomnia
I. Anorexia—causes in the older adult
 1. Forgetting to eat
 2. Side effects of drugs
 3. Gum disease
 4. Dentures
J. Substance abuse—most common categories
 1. Prescription drugs
    a. Diazepam (Valium)
    b. Chlordiazepoxide (Librium)
    c. Prochlorperazine (Compazine)
 2. Over-the-counter drugs
    a. Aspirin
    b. Laxatives
    c. Antacids
 3. Alcohol
    a. Abused throughout life
    b. Use may be in response to aging
    c. Intermittent use in response to stress
    d. Drink because of
       (1) Loss

(2) Loneliness

(3) Illness

   e. Contributes to falls and accidents

K. **Isolation and loneliness**

   1. Loneliness—reactive response to separation from persons and things of significance; may result in isolation of self from others

   2. Causative factors of loneliness and isolation in the older adult

      a. Death of a spouse

      b. Loss of bodily functions

      c. Loss of sensory acuity

      d. Death, relocation, or physical illness of a sibling, neighbor, or roommate

      e. Loss of a pet

      f. Geographic move

      g. Language barriers

      h. Lowered energy levels

      i. Pain

      j. Changes in body image

      k. Economic changes

      l. Organic problems

      m. Eccentricity

      n. Structural barriers

   (Modified from Haber et al, 1992)

III. Common losses experienced by the older adult (one or more of these losses may result in a bereavement response) (Clinical Example 17-1)

A. Self-care ability

B. Independence

C. Vision

Clinical Example 17-1. Bereavement Response

Client is a 73-year-old caucasian, widowed female. She is admitted to the emergency room with a 20-pound weight loss over the last 2 months, difficulty falling asleep, and lack of interest in attending any social events related to her senior group. She states that life is not really worth living at this point. Her husband died 3 months earlier. They had been married 50 years and have two children and eight grandchildren, who all live out of state. She and her husband had regularly attended senior group activities together. Her husband always drove to activities, as the client has no driver's license. Since his death, the client has remained at home and has attended no activities other than church. She is brought to the emergency room by her pastor.

    D. Hearing

    E. Mobility

    F. Health

    G. Memory

    H. Intellect

    I. Work

    J. Financial security

    K. Family and friends

    L. Personal possessions

    M. Sense of belonging

    N. Sense of purpose

    O. Meaning in Life

    (Modified from Haber et al, 1992)

IV. Application of the nursing process with the older adult

    A. Assessment

        1. Select a quiet setting—older adults have diminished high-frequency hearing

        2. Speak slowly in a low-pitched voice

        3. Assess for limitations in mobility

            a. Wheelchairs

            b. Walkers

            c. Orthostatic hypotension

        4. Assess for problems with nutrition

            a. Visual problems preparing food

            b. Loss of teeth or chewing ability

            c. Problems with swallowing include types of food eaten or shortness of breath

            d. Periodontal disease

        5. Mental status

            a. Mental status questionnaire (MSQ)—10 mental status questions about

                (1) Place

                (2) Date

                (3) Day of week

                (4) Age

                (5) Birth date

            b. Short portable mental status questionnaire (SPMSQ)—assesses

                (1) Orientation

                (2) Remote memory

                (3) Recent memory

        (4)   Math ability

        (5)   Practical skills

  c. Face-hand test

        (1)   Tests for organicity

        (2)   Recognize tactile stimulation on cheek and back of hand

        (3)   Do a sequence of touching right and left cheek and back of each hand

  d. Mini-mental state examination—assesses

        (1)   Orientation

        (2)   Attention

        (3)   Calculations

        (4)   Recall (repeating three objects named earlier)

        (5)   Language (write a sentence)

        (6)   Cognitive functioning

  e. Zung self-rative depression scale—assesses for risk of depression

        (1)   10 negative items

        (2)   10 positive items

        (3)   Clients rate with likert scale format how often item happens to them

      (Modified from Stuart and Sundeen, 1995)

6. Activities of daily living—assessment tools

  a. Katz index of activities of daily living—rates ability of client to perform six functions independently

        (1)   Bathing

        (2)   Dressing

        (3)   Toileting

        (4)   Transfer

        (5)   Continence

        (6)   Feeding

  b. Pace II

        (1)   Facilitates the evaluation of physical health of nursing home patients

        (2)   Checklist

        (3)   Duration, type, and location of problem are identified

7. Family interaction—assessment tools

  a. Family apgar—each family member rates the family in categories and results indicates dysfunction in the family

        (1)   Partnership

              (2) Affection

              (3) Growth

      b. Social behavior assessment schedule—use of significant other to collect information on client's social functioning

              (1) Withdrawal

              (2) Forgetfulness

              (3) Indecisiveness

              (4) Household tasks

B. Nursing diagnoses

    1. Altered thought process

      a. Memory loss

      b. Confusion

          (1) Sunrise

          (2) Sundown

      c. Paranoia

    2. Social isolation

    3. Dysfunctional grieving

      a. Depression

      b. Sadness

      c. Prolonged grief

      d. Fatigue

      e. Anorexia

      f. Apathy

      g. Loss of interest

      h. Psychomotor retardation

      i. Attitudes to own death

    4. Sleep pattern disturbance

      a. Interrupted sleep

      b. Morning exhaustion

      c. Becomes cyclical process—worry over lack of sleep

    5. Altered nutrition—less than body requirements

C. Goals for older clients

    1. Client will maintain optimal level of autonomy

    2. Client will participate in activities of daily living

    3. Client will maintain adequate nutrition

    4. Client will have adequate sleep without fatigue

    5. Client will not experience signs of clinical depression related to various losses

    6. Client will not be exposed to dangerous situations as a result of altered thought process

    7. Client will interact socially with peers via social clubs, scheduled activities, social outings

    8. Client will review life and experience a sense of dignity

D. **Nursing interventions**
1. Life review therapy
    a. Reflect on life
    b. Resolve, reorganize, integrate disturbing areas
    c. Done in groups or individually
    d. Encourage expression of feelings and meanings related to the content being presented
    e. Result—sense of integrity and integration with life
2. Reminiscing groups
    a. Recount earlier life experiences
    b. Share experiences of a historical (WWII) or personal event
3. Reality orientation
    a. Environment—provide
        (1) Clocks
        (2) Signs
        (3) Calendars
        (4) Orientation boards with seasons and next holiday
    b. Groups—reinforce time, place, person
4. Validation therapy—focus on feelings and meanings with the confused client versus reorientation
5. Cognitive training
    a. "Use it or lose it"
    b. Memory exercises
    c. Intelligence does not decline with age
    d. Problem-solving situations are used
6. Relaxation therapy—relaxation with mild exercise increases cardiovascular output and energy
    (Modified from Stuart and Sundeen, 1995)
E. **Evaluation**
1. Client participates in own care as physical and emotional limitations allow
2. Client sleeps 6 to 7 hours per night and reports minimal fatigue
3. Client verbalizes feelings related to multiple losses in life and displays no signs of depression
4. Client participates in life review groups, reality orientation groups, and reminiscing groups and shares experiences and feelings in group
5. Client experiences a sense of dignity in the life review process

REVIEW QUESTIONS

1. A depressed older-adult client is more often treated with desipramine (Norpramine) because it
   a. Has a low anticholinergic effect
   b. Has fewer adverse reactions with other drugs
   c. Has a significant sedative property
   d. Is effective if given in small doses

2. In which diagnosis can a living will be considered valid to give directions to healthcare providers?
   a. Alzheimer's disease
   b. Dementia
   c. Antisocial personality
   d. Terminal carcinoma

3. During evaluation of an older-adult client's memory, the use of reminiscences is helpful because
   a. The client will feel more relaxed
   b. The client will feel more positive
   c. Memory chains are stimulated
   d. Judgment and intellect can be evaluated

4. In a presentation to a group of clients living independently in a complex for persons over 60, the nurse might want to include which factor as most commonly leading to accidents in older adults?
   a. Inability to maintain sensory acuity
   b. Decreased mobility
   c. Impaired mobility
   d. Short-term memory loss

5. The nurse admits a 92-year-old client with cluster bruises on the trunk, welts on the lower legs, and highly odorous clothing. The client withdrew and looked away when the nurse applied the blood pressure cuff. After the initial physical assessment, what is the nurse's next best action?
   a. Notify the physician of possible abuse
   b. Contact social services to initiate an investigation for possible abuse
   c. Document the observations and indicators of mistreatment
   d. Explore with the client further for establishment of mistreatment

ANSWERS, RATIONALES, AND TEST-TAKING TIPS

Rationales	Test-Taking Tips

1. Correct answer: a

This becomes a drug of choice for older adults because they are susceptible to anticholinergic side effects such as decreased peristalsis, increased urine retention, and decreased secretions.

For this type of difficult question, make your best educated guess, take three deep breaths with your eyes closed, and proceed to the next question. The important thing is not to get emotionally upset and to maintain your clear thinking for the remainder of the questions.

2. Correct answer: d

Living wills are valid only in diagnoses of terminal illness. Living wills do not extend to disorders of cognitive functioning.

Cluster the options that interfere with normal functioning of the mind and select option *d,* which typically does not affect the mind.

3. Correct answer: c

Reminiscence and reminiscence groups are very helpful in stimulating the older adult's memory by attempting to recall patterns of association that will improve recall and recollection.

If you have no idea of the correct answer, simply match the theme of the question—assessment of memory—with the option that has memory in it, *c.*

4. Correct answer: c

The most common factor in accidents is impaired mobility. Sensory function is diminished, and the client has no ability to maintain the sensory functions. Decreased mobility lends itself to constipation and venous stasis. Memory function has nothing to do with accident frequency.

The best approach is to eliminate options based on what you know about the relationship between normal decreased functions in the older adult and accidents. The other important part is to read the options closely to identify what makes them incorrect.

5. **Correct answer: c**

The nurse should document the information as soon as possible after collection to be the most accurate. After that, the sequence of actions might be options *d, a,* then *b.*

The key words are "after the initial assessment . . . the next best action." Document, do further assessment, then lastly notify appropriate authorities.

Organic Mental Disorders

STUDY OUTCOMES

After completing this chapter, the reader will be able to do the following:

▼ Identify major theories related to the etiology of dementia.

▼ Define cognition.

▼ Discuss predisposing factors related to cognitive disorders.

▼ Describe precipitating stressors that contribute to cognitive disorders.

▼ Differentiate between the behaviors of an individual with delirium and one with dementia.

▼ Describe the purposes of several psychological tests.

▼ Identify coping mechanisms used by clients with cognitive disorders.

▼ Apply the nursing process with a client experiencing a cognitive disorder.

KEY TERMS

Agnosia	Total or partial loss of the ability to recognize familiar objects or persons through sensory stimuli (Rawlins et al, 1993).
Amnestic disorder	Memory impairment in the absence of other significant cognitive impairments.
Anomia	Inability to remember names and objects (Haber et al, 1992).
Aphasia	Loss of ability to use meaningful speech.
Apraxia	Inability to understand the meaning of things (Haber et al, 1992).
Confabulation	The manufacture of a response that is inaccurate but sounds appropriate; done in an effort to cover up memory loss (Stuart and Sundeen, 1995).
Delirium	Disturbance of consciousness and cognitive impairments with an acute onset and with the identification of a specific precipitating stressor; is usually reversible when treated.
Dementia	Multiple cognitive impairments that are usually gradual in onset and irreversible.
Organic disorder	Mental or emotional impairment believed to be physiological in origin.
Paraphasia	Misuse of spoken words or word combinations (Haber et al, 1992).

CONTENT REVIEW

I. Cognition
A. Definition
1. The ability to think and reason; cognition includes the processes of
   a. Memory
   b. Judgement
   c. Orientation
   d. Perception
   e. Attention
B. Cognitive impairment
1. A state of confusion
2. Unable to understand experiences
3. Unable to relate current to past events

    4. Unable to make decisions

    5. A frightening experience

II. Predisposing factors to cognitive disorders

  A. **Biological factors**

    1. Interruption in nutrients to brain

      a. Transient ischemia attacks

      b. Cerebral hemorrhage

      c. Multiple small infarcts (chronic hypertension)

    2. Degeneration of brain tissue (aging)

    3. Toxic chemicals or heavy metals

    4. Metabolic disorders

      a. Chronic renal disease

      b. Vitamin deficiencies

        (1) Vitamin B complex

        (2) Thiamine

      c. Malnutrition

    5. Alcoholism

    6. Korsakoff's psychosis

    7. Wernicke's syndrome

    8. AIDS-related dementia

  B. **Genetic**

    1. Huntington's chorea—autosomal dominant trait

    2. Alzheimer's disease theory

    3. Down syndrome

  C. **Disruption in mental functioning**

    1. Delusions

    2. Short attention span

    3. Depression—memory disorders

III. Precipitating stressors to cognitive disorders

  A. **Hypoxia**

    1. Chronic obstructive pulmonary disease

    2. Anemia from occult bleeding

    3. Deficiencies

      a. Iron

      b. Folic acid

      c. Vitamin B_{12}

    4. Asthma

    5. Acute respiratory tract infection

    6. Congestive heart failure

    7. Atherosclerosis

      8. Hypotension
      9. Hypertension
  B. **Metabolic disorders**
      1. Hypothyroidism—retarded in thinking
      2. Hyperthyroidism—delusional thinking
      3. Hypoglycemia
      4. Hypopituitarism
      5. Adrenal disease
  C. **Toxic and infectious agents**
      1. Increased urea levels—renal failure
      2. Toxic wastes
      3. Animal venoms
      4. Tertiary syphilis
      5. Human immunodeficiency virus type I (HIV-I)
      6. Drug interactions
  D. **Structural changes**
      1. Tumors
      2. Trauma
  E. **Sensory overstimulation or understimulation—"ICU psychosis"**

IV. Types of cognitive disorders

  A. **Delirium (Table 18-1)**
      1. Clouding of awareness
      2. Limited attention span
      3. Sensory misperception
         a. Illusions—a dot on the wall is perceived as a spider
         b. Hallucinations
            (1) Visual—animals, reptiles, insects
            (2) Frightening to clients
      4. Disordered thought process
         a. Disturbed attention
         b. Memory impairment
         c. Disoriented in all three spheres
         d. Poor judgement
         e. Little decision-making ability
      5. Change in activity pattern
         a. Assaultive behavior
         b. Destructive behavior
      6. Labile affect—tearful then laughing in a few minutes
      7. Loss of appropriate social behavior
         a. Undress in public
         b. Grab at people
         c. Play with food

Table 18-1. **Characteristics of Delirium and Dementia**

Factor	Delirium	Dementia
Onset	Usually sudden	Usually gradual
Course	Usually brief (under 1 month), with return to usual level of functioning	Usually long term and progressive; occasionally may be arrested or reversed
Age Group	Any	Most common over age 65
Stressors	Toxins, infection, hyperthermia, space-occupying lesion, trauma, and sensory deprivation/overload	Hypertension, hypotension, anemia, normal pressure hydrocephalus, vitamin deficiencies, toxins, slow viruses, hypoglycemia, tumors, hyperthermia/ hypothermia, and brain tissue atrophy
Behaviors	Fluctuating levels of awareness, disorientation, restlessness, agitation, illusions, hallucinations, disorganized thought, impaired judgement and decision making, affective lability, loss of inhibitions, and diffuse electroencephalogram (EEG) slowing	Memory loss, impaired judgement, decreased attention span, disorientation, inappropriate social behavior, labile affect, restlessness, agitation, and resistance to change

Stuart G and Sundeen S: *Principles and practice of psychiatric nursing,* ed 4, St Louis, 1991, Mosby.

8. Impulsive
9. Symptoms fluctuate throughout the day—intermittently lucid
10. Physiological causes of delirium
    a. Infection
    b. Trauma
    c. Drug or alcohol intoxication
11. Rapid onset of symptoms
12. Usually brief
13. May progress to dementia if untreated
B. **Dementia**
    1. Loss of intellectual ability
       a. Memory

      b. Judgement

      c. Abstract thought

  2. Changes in personality

      a. Alteration of personality

      b. Accentuation of usual character traits

  3. Disorientation—time lost first, then place, then person

  4. Memory loss

      a. Recent memory lost first

      b. Confabulate

          (1) Make up information to fill in memory gaps

          (2) Used to save embarrassment

  5. Labile effect

  6. Impulsive sexual behavior

  7. Decreased inhibition

  8. Restlessness

  9. Agitation—sundown syndrome

  10. Onset usually gradual

  11. Can be reversed if cause is identified and treated; otherwise is irreversible

  12. Most often occurs in older adults

  13. Causes of dementia

      a. Trauma

      b. Chronic infection—tertiary syphilis

      c. Arteriosclerosis

      d. Chronic hypertension

  14. Seven types of dementia

      a. Alzheimer's disease (Clinical Example 18-1)

          (1) Atrophy of the cortex

Clinical Example 18-1. Alzheimer's Disease

The client is a 74-year-old caucasian, widowed female. Over the last 2 years she has had increasing difficulty with her memory. Initially she experienced difficulty in driving her car. She could not locate places with which she had in the past been quite familiar. As time progressed, the client was unable to continue driving, as she was often lost and unable to find her way home. Additionally, she would find herself in the middle of a conversation and forget what the topic was. She compensated for this by making up a topic (confabulation). Managing her diabetes became difficult in terms of remembering insulin doses and times for blood testing. She is diagnosed with early stages of Alzheimer's disease.

Modified from Stuart G, and Sundeen S: *Principles and practice of psychiatric nursing,* ed 4, St Louis, 1991, Mosby.

(2) Plaques and fluid pockets in the hippocampus—the center for short-term memory
(3) Deficiency of neurotransmitter—acetylcholine
(4) Stages of symptoms
    (a) Stage one
        (i) Memory loss caused by patchy loss of neurons throughout the cerebral cortex
        (ii) Judgement and logic compensate for memory deficits
        (iii) As the disease progresses, judgement and logic decline
        (iv) Disorientation and global aphasia occur
            ▼ Broca's aphasia—motor and expressive speech deficits
            ▼ Wernicke's aphasia—sensory comprehension deficits
        (v) Irritability
        (vi) Mood swings
        (vii) Flattening of affect
        (viii) Agitation
    (b) Stage two: 2 to 4 years into the disease
        (i) Increased loss of frontal and temporal lobe function
        (ii) Forget learned, socially acceptable behaviors
        (iii) Neglect hygiene
        (iv) Develop inappropriate eating habits
        (v) Poor elimination patterns
        (vi) Lose portions of ability to see, hear, and feel pain
        (vii) Agnosia
        (viii) May have seizures
        (ix) Perseveration—repetition of a motor or verbal action
        (x) Hyperorality—insatiable need for oral stimulation by chewing or tasting objects
        (xi) This stage lasts 2 to 12 years
        (xii) Regression is more rapid in younger people and in men
    (c) Stage three
        (i) Impaired, confusional stage
        (ii) Progression of generalized and focal deficits

        (iii) Unresponsive

        (iv) Anorexia

        (v) Apraxia—an impairment in the ability to perform purposeful acts or to manipulate objects. Types of apraxia

            ▼ Ideation—loss of the perception of the use of an object

            ▼ Motor—inability to use an object or perform a task without loss of perception of the use of the object or the goal of the task

            ▼ Speech—inability to program the position of speech muscles and the sequence of muscle movement necessary to produce understandable speech

            ▼ Amnestic—inability to perform the function because of an inability to remember the command to perform it

  b. Vascular dementia

      1. Disruptions in cerebral blood supply

      2. Thrombi, emboli

      3. Infarction of brain tissue

  c. Dementia related to HIV disease

      (1) Destruction of white matter and subcortical structures

      (2) Forgetfulness

      (3) Slowness

      (4) Poor concentration

      (5) Apathy

      (6) Social withdrawal

      (7) Delusions

      (8) Hallucinations

      (9) Tremors

      (10) Ataxia

      (11) Hypertonia

      (12) Hyperreflexia

  d. Parkinson's disease

      (1) A neurological condition from a deficiency in dopamine—a dysfunction in the basal ganglia

      (2) Nonintentional tremor—"pill rolling" of fingers

            (3)   Rigidity of muscle movement

            (4)   Memory impairment

     e.   Huntington's disease

            (1)   Genetic—autosomal dominant gene

            (2)   Progressive

            (3)   Degenerative in areas of

               (a)   Cognition

               (b)   Emotion

               (c)   Movement

            (4)   Depression

            (5)   Irritability

            (6)   Anxiety

     f.   Pick's disease

            (1)   Degeneration of frontal and temporal lobes

            (2)   Personality changes

            (3)   Deterioration of social skills

            (4)   Blunting of affect

            (5)   Loss of memory

            (6)   Apraxia

     g.   Substance-induced, persisting dementia

            (1)   Memory impairment

            (2)   Aphasia

            (3)   Apraxia

            (4)   Agnosia

            (5)   Problems with abstract thinking

C. Amnestic disorders

    1.   Definition—disturbance in memory

       a.   Related to a medical condition

       b.   Related to effects of a substance

            (1)   Drug

            (2)   Toxin

            (3)   Medication

    2.   Unable to learn new information

    3.   Unable to recall previously learned information

    4.   Common causes

       a.   Stroke

       b.   Carbon monoxide poisoning

       c.   Prolonged substance abuse

            (1)   Chronic alcoholism

            (2)   Wernicke-Korsakoff's syndrome

       d.   Nutritional deficiency

       e.   Head trauma

V. Psychological testing
A. Purposes
1. Identifying of stressors causing disorder
2. Understanding dynamics of the problem
3. Developing plan for interventions
4. Establishing prognosis

B. Types (Table 18-2)

Table 18-2. Types of Personality Tests

Type	Purpose	Results
Intelligence		
Wechsler Intelligence Scale for Children (WISC) (for children only) Wechsler Adult Intelligence Scale (WAIS)	Assess general level of intellectual functioning	Intelligence Quotient (IQ) Guideline for understanding intellectual ability
Perceptual-motor testing		
Bender-Gestalt Test	Determine if an organic problem is causing disturbed behavior	Accuracy and ability to copy geometrical figures determine presence of biological problems
Projective Tests		
Rorscharch Test	Both: Gain information about psychodynamics	Responses to inkblots are analyzed
Thematic Apperception Test (TAT)		Client describes drawings of people engaged in nonspecific activities Information is gained on the anxiety level of coping mechanisms

Modified from Stuart G, and Sundeen S: *Principles and practice of psychiatric nursing*, ed 4, St Louis, 1991, Mosby.

VI. Coping mechanisms utilized by clients with cognitive disorders

A. Ways of coping are related to past experience
B. Response to the disease relates to past personality
1. Repression of anger-depression
2. Anger toward others
C. Regression
1. More dependent on others
2. Deterioration in mental function
D. Denial
1. Attempts to pursue usual routine
2. Makes light of memory problems
3. Utilizes people around him or her to help with memory problems
E. Suspiciousness
F. Hostility
G. Joking
H. Seductiveness
I. Withdrawal
(Modified from Stuart and Sundeen, 1995)

VII. Application of the nursing process with the client experiencing a cognitive disorder

A. Nursing assessment
1. Abstract thinking and reasoning—ask client for similarities and differences between objects
   a. Bus–Train
   b. Window–Door
   c. Dog–Goldfish
2. Judgement and decision making
   a. "What would you do with a stamped, addressed envelope?"
   b. "What would you do if you were in a theater and a fire broke out?"
3. Calculations—count backward from 100 in increments of 7
4. General knowledge
   a. "Who is the president of the United States?"
   b. "What are the names of the oceans?"
5. Ability to comprehend new knowledge—abnormal responses indicate cognitive disorder
   a. Cannot verbalize four unrelated words after 5 minutes (example: girl, red, window, car)
   b. Cannot remember an address 5 minutes after it is given

6. Recent memory
   a. "How long have you been here?"
   b. "What did you have for breakfast today?"
7. Lack of insight
   a. "Why did you decide to come to the hospital at this time?"
   b. "Have you noticed any changes in yourself?"
8. Apresia—assess ability to communicate thoughts in speech, writing, or symbols
9. Agnosia
   a. Ask them to identify objects
   b. Check for recognition of significant others
10. Apraxia—observe for ability to utilize familiar tools
    a. Silverware
    b. Razor
11. Perseveration—assess for repetition of words
12. Obsessive-compulsive behaviors
    a. "Have you ever had a thought that you couldn't get rid of?"
    b. "Have you ever had to complete a task despite feedback that it was time to change the plan?"
    c. "Do you ever have to perform an act to decrease your anxiety?"
13. Delusional content
    a. "Have you ever felt you were being watched or singled out?"
    b. "Have you ever felt as if you were being controlled by external forces?"
    c. "Have you ever felt that you have overwhelming powers?"
    d. "Have you ever been preoccupied with a part of your body or felt that it was malfunctioning in some way?"
    e. "Have you ever felt as if you were detached from your body?"

B. **Nursing diagnoses**
   1. Alteration in sensory perception
   2. Altered health maintenance
   3. Altered role performance
   4. Altered thought process
   5. Anxiety
   6. Bowel incontinence
   7. Diversional activity deficit
   8. Fear
   9. Impaired home maintenance management
   10. Impaired physical mobility

11. Impaired social interaction
12. Impaired verbal communication
13. Ineffective family coping
14. Ineffective individual coping
15. Risk for injury
16. Risk for trauma
17. Self-care deficit
18. Sleep pattern disturbance
19. Social isolation
20. Withdrawal

C. **Goals for client**
1. Client will demonstrate an intellect and judgement to the best of ability based on cognitive functioning
2. Client will reminisce about past life experiences using long-term memory functions
3. Client will respond coherently to simple, concrete statements
4. Client will demonstrate absence of overt anxiety, fear, and confusion
5. Client will follow concrete directions
6. Client will participate in basic decisions about activities of daily living, such as selecting clothing and deciding on a menu
7. Client will be oriented to person, place, time, and situation
8. Client will maintain residual sensory-perceptual functions
(Modified from Fortinash and Holoday-Worret, 1991)

D. **Nursing interventions (Table 18-3)**

E. **Evaluation of client**
1. Client is able to make decisions related to activities of daily living, such as choosing a menu and selecting clothes
2. Client is willing to discuss past life experiences with staff and other clients
3. Client is able to appropriately respond to simple questions from staff
4. Client is not displaying signs and symptoms of anxiety or fear
5. Client is oriented to person, place, time, and situation
6. Client participates in unit activities such as music therapy, and exercise group
7. Client is able to follow simple directions from staff
8. Client is not delusional, experiencing hallucinations, or easily redirected
(Modified from Fortinash and Holloday-Worret, 1991).

Table 18-3. Nursing Interventions for the Cognitively Impaired with Appropriate Rationales

Intervention	Rationale
Identify yourself and look directly into client's eyes	Need to have nurse's identity established. If you don't have the client's attention, the client will misinterpret your words and become confused and frightened.
Speak to the client in a clear, low-pitched voice	High-pitched tones create anxiety and tension in clients with cognitive disorders
When speaking to the client, eliminate distracting background stimuli such as radio, television, and extraneous talking	Too much stimulation results in sensory overload and confuses the client
Ask only one question at a time with the use of short, simple sentences	Decreases confusion, promotes concentration, and increases attention span
Repeat the question if the client does not respond or does not seem to understand your meaning. Use the same words.	Repetition reinforces comprehension. Changing the words will further confuse the client.
Use "yes" or "no" questions whenever possible, and avoid those that require choices for making decisions	Clients cannot make complex decisions and will only feel frustrated when confronted with such a task
Break down tasks into individual steps and ask the client to do one step at a time	Clients cannot tend to more than one task or step at a time
Use strategies to promote REM (rapid eye movement) sleep ▼ Allow client to walk in a secure area during the day ▼ Eliminate or reduce daytime naps ▼ Engage client in an active daily schedule	REM sleep promotes rest and prevents confusion, disorientation, and irritability
Increase stimulation if the client appears restless or confused or wanders during the night. Use ▼ Lights ▼ Soft music	Clients who are suddenly deprived of routine daily activities require some stimulation to prevent restlessness and promote sleep

Table 18-3. Nursing Interventions for the Cognitively Impaired with Appropriate Rationales—cont'd

Intervention	Rationale
Arrange the unit with a reality-orientation board that includes easy-to-read clock, calendar, menu, name of facility, and city and state	To enhance optimal memory function, orientation, and thought processes
In the client's room, place familiar and cherished objects such as family photographs, pet pictures, and quilts	Promotes comfort and enhances memory function
Maintain routine and structure within the unit	Clients have a difficult time coping with changes in routine
Use pictures to communicate with clients who have aphasia	To enhance understanding of the meaning of the message
Initiate a pet therapy session	To produce a calming effect; promote comfort, love, and affection; enhance the senses; and support memory function
Engage in reminiscence sessions by reviewing past experiences such as by looking through photo albums	To utilize functional remote memory and promote feelings of enjoyment and belonging
Reassure and comfort a client who seems lost and confused. Inform the client about where he or she is, why, and for how long.	To decrease fear and anxiety related to feelings of abandonment or confusion
Refrain from confronting or arguing with a suspicious or paranoid client. Redirect to another activity.	Pursuing the belief may promote agitation or aggression
Refrain from agreeing with confabulation; instead, gently correct the person rather than try to convince him or her that he or she is wrong	Decreases anxiety and prevents embarrassment
Refrain from agreeing or disagreeing with the validity of a client's delusion; instead, respond to the feeling that the client demonstrates	Denying or confirming a fixed belief will only increase confusion and anxiety
Use humor when feasible	Humor is a universal language that enhances communication and social interactions

Continued.

Table 18-3. Nursing Interventions for the Cognitively Impaired with Appropriate Rationales—cont'd

Intervention	Rationale
Ignore crude or vulgar remarks; instead, assess the intent behind the words or activity	Clients occasionally lose ability to control socially inappropriate behaviors
Assist the client with basic care and personal hygiene needs	To promote comfort, build self-esteem, and protect from ridicule
Engage the client in interactive therapies such as music, stretching exercises, and cooking	To increase involvement and interpersonal interactions with staff and other clients
Administer antipsychotic medication as necessary. Haldol is common.	To reduce agitation and prevent escalation of behaviors that may be harmful
Gently restrain the client if he or she cannot be distracted and behavior escalates to an unmanageable level.	To protect the client and others from harm or injury

Modified from Fortinash K and Holloday-Worret P: *Psychiatric nursing care plans,* St Louis, 1991, Mosby.

REVIEW QUESTIONS

1. Which is inappropriate to use as a basis to suspect dementia?
   a. Impairment in short-term memory
   b. Transient confusion
   c. Impairment in long-term memory
   d. Significant changes in social relationships

2. Alzheimer's disease is primarily characterized by
   a. Progressive memory decline
   b. Emotional disturbances
   c. Dysphoria
   d. Hallucinations

3. A client with dementia is noted to have a disorder of language. This may be documented as
   a. Agnosia
   b. Anhedonia
   c. Apraxia
   d. Aphasia

4. A client is diagnosed with irreversible dementia. During the initial assessment, this client's intellectual abilities would most likely reveal
   a. Impaired long-term memory
   b. Intact short-term memory
   c. Disorientation to time and place
   d. Inability to communicate

5. The client with irreversible dementia talks about the younger days and occasionally confabulates. Confabulation means
   a. The loss of the ability to speak
   b. The continuous repetition of words
   c. The tendency to relate imaginary experiences to fill in memory gaps
   d. The inability to recognize one's own life experiences

6. In planning care for a client with irreversible dementia, what is most essential?
   a. Firmness
   b. Detailed explanations
   c. Nutritional needs
   d. Consistency

ANSWERS, RATIONALES, AND TEST-TAKING TIPS

Rationales	Test-Taking Tips

1. **Correct answer: b**

   Transient confusion is not a symptom of dementia. Abstract thinking, impaired judgement, aphasia, apraxia, agnosia, and personality changes are seen and used in the diagnosis after physiologic causes are ruled out.

   The important approach is to read the question correctly. If you read too fast, are tense or tired, you may miss the key word, "inappropriate."

2. **Correct answer: a**

   Alzheimer's disease is a deterioration in all areas of cognitive functioning, including changes in memory, personality, mood, and behavior. Dysphoria is a disturbance of affect characterized by depression and anguish. Hallucination is a perceptual distortion arising from any of the five senses.

   The key words are "primarily characterized by." In narrowing the responses to *a* and *b*—a memory or an emotional problem—*go with what you know,* that Alzheimer's is progressive memory loss.

3. **Correct answer: d**

   Aphasia is a deficit in the spoken and/or written language; more specifically, in Alzheimer's aphasia is characterized as difficulty in finding the right word. The client's language may become vague and imprecise. In the final stages of Alzhiemer's, language and the ability to speak may be lost entirely. Agnosia is difficulty in recognizing well-known objects. Anhedonia is an

   Go with what you know if you have no idea of the correct answer. Associate language problems with stroke clients who have either expressive or receptive aphasia. Identify the clue in the stem, "language," and select option *d.*

inability or decreased ability to experience pleasure, joy, intimacy, and closeness. Apraxia is inability to perform familiar skilled activities.

4. **Correct answer: c**

When clients with this diagnosis are placed in new or unfamiliar surroundings, they become easily confused and disoriented. The other responses are incorrect for the given information.

The clue in the stem is the word "initial" for the assessment. Eliminate options *a* and *b,* since with the diagnosis of irreversible dementia the client most likely has both memories impaired. With options *c* and *d* left, there is more likely an orientation problem on initial assessment.

5. **Correct answer: c**

Confabulation is the fabrication of experiences or events, often recalled in detail to cover for gaps in memory.

Associate confabulation with fables or stories that are fabulated or made up.

6. **Correct answer: d**

Consistency in the care of these clients is needed to provide a known routine and to reduce confusion.

The clue to option *d* is "when planning care," which is a general focus. Option *a* is a general option but being firm may cause these clients to become irritated and hostile. Remember that consistency provides comfort in most clinical situations. Eliminate option *c,* since nutrition is too narrow of a response. Detailed explanations are inappropriate; simplicity is the better approach with these clients.

Comprehensive
Exam

COMPREHENSIVE EXAM QUESTIONS

1. What is the primary difference between a social and therapeutic relationship?
   a. The amount of emotion invested
   b. The degree of satisfaction attained
   c. The kind of information given
   d. The type of responsibility involved

2. A nurse evaluates that a client, after 5 days on the voluntary psychiatric unit, returns to the behavior, modes of gratification, and adaptation of a person much younger. This would be documented as
   a. Rationalization
   b. Regression
   c. Repression
   d. Suppression

3. After a telephone conversation, a client in a voluntary psychiatric unit seems agitated and restless. The client stares out the window and appears upset. When the nurse questions the client, he states, "I don't want to discuss anything right now." The defense mechanism manifested by this behavior is
   a. Suppression
   b. Sublimation
   c. Substitution
   d. Symbolization

4. A man is in danger of losing his job. He decides to go on a cruise and consciously not think about work so his trip won't be spoiled. This is an example of
   a. Regression
   b. Denial
   c. Suppression
   d. Repression

5. Which defense mechanism may be more commonly considered fully compatible with mental health?
   a. Isolation
   b. Sublimation
   c. Regression
   d. Projection

6. In which type of meeting are client behaviors discussed individually, with decisions made about treatments?
   a. Group meetings
   b. Community meetings
   c. Team meetings
   d. Supervision meetings

7. Clients admitted involuntarily to a mental health clinic have had their status changed to a voluntary admission. This means the clients can now
   a. Receive personal mail and visitors
   b. Speak to the client advocate
   c. Refuse treatment
   d. Request to see an attorney

8. Which situation would be a breach in the confidentiality of a client?
   a. A nursing student looking at the chart of a client not assigned to the student's care
   b. A nurse documenting the behavior of the client
   c. A nurse discussing the client's behavior with his family
   d. A nurse discussing the client's behavior with the client's employer

9. A client on the unit believes another client has stolen his watch, and they want to discuss this with the nurse. What is the nurse's best response?
   a. "I'll meet with each of you individually"
   b. "Tell me what you believed happened"
   c. "I'm sure no one here would do a thing like that"
   d. "Be careful when you accuse someone"

10. The nurse is discussing the orientation phase. The student nurse asks what the primary goal between the nurse and the client is during this phase. The nurse should respond that the primary goal is to
    a. Explain unit rules
    b. Establish a relationship
    c. Establish trust and rapport
    d. Formulate a mutual plan of action

11. A nurse is talking with a client who is hearing voices. The nurse states, "The only voices I hear are yours and mine." This is an example of
    a. Restating
    b. Clarification
    c. Focusing
    d. Presenting reality

12. A client is scheduled for surgery. Which of the following statements by the nurse would most likely encourage the client to verbalize feelings about the impending surgery?
    a. "Everything will be all right"
    b. "Things have a way of working out"
    c. "This must be a difficult time for you"
    d. "Your physician is very competent"

13. During ECT the client might be expected to
    a. Have a partial seizure
    b. Have a tonic-clonic seizure
    c. Have a multiple seizure
    d. Have a general seizure

14. A nurse is caring for a client with schizophrenia. What medication would the nurse expect the client to be receiving?
    a. Buspirone (Buspar)
    b. Chlorpromazine (Thorazine)
    c. Lithium carbonate (Lithium)
    d. Fluoxetine (Prozac)

15. A client has been medicated with trifluperazine HCL (Stelazine) for a prolonged period of time. How would the nurse check for early signs of tardive dyskinesia?
    a. Akathisia of the lower extremities
    b. Cogwheel rigidity at the elbow
    c. Drying of the mucous membranes
    d. Vermiform movements of the tongue

16. When the nurse checks the lithium level of a client on the unit, it is 2.0 mEq/L. What should the interpretation/action by the nurse be?
    a. The level is within therapeutic range; do nothing
    b. The level is below therapeutic range; call the physician
    c. The level is slightly elevated but does not require any nursing action
    d. This level is high; the client should be assessed for manifestations of toxicity

17. A client's wife approaches the nurse with questions regarding her husband's medications. He is now on day 5 of taking his antidepressant and, as his wife states, "He is no better; I just don't see any improvement." What is the nurse's best response?
    a. "Try not to worry. Things will get better in 3 to 4 months."
    b. "Antidepressants take longer than other medications to work"

    c. "Most antidepressants take 2 to 4 weeks before any effect of the medication is seen"

    d. "I know this is upsetting, but I've seen antidepressants work well with other clients over a period of just a few more weeks"

18. Which antipsychotic, when given IM, is stored in the fat and released slowly into the blood to provide extended action?
    a. Chlorpromazine HCl (Thorazine)
    b. Loxopine HCl (Loxitane)
    c. Fluphenazine deconate (Prolixin Deconate)
    d. Trifluoperazine HCl (Stelazine)

19. Which antidepressant would the nurse expect to administer to treat depression, severe obsessive-compulsive disorder (the primary diagnosis), and phobic disorder?
    a. Phenelzine sulfate (Nardil)
    b. Clomipramine (Anafranil)
    c. Amitriptyline HCl (Elavil)
    d. Imipramine (Tofranil)

20. The client is on propanalol (Inderal), an antianxiety agent. What is most important to include in the teaching plan?
    a. Take the medication at the same time everyday
    b. Few differences exist among antianxiety agents
    c. Drug dosages are often titrated
    d. These medications should be used during a period of specific stress

21. On the morning of ECT, the client is to receive atropine gr 1/150 IM before treatment. On hand is atropine 0.4 mg/ml. How much atropine will the nurse administer?
    a. 1.0 ml
    b. 0.5 ml
    c. 0.75 ml
    d. 1.5 ml

22. Which statement offered by a nurse best defines the aim of structured groups?
    a. "These groups serve an essential need and provide support"
    b. "This type of group provides members with awareness of some of life's problems and tools to cope"
    c. "This group has a focus on the group process rather than on personal growth"
    d. "This group process offers intense experiences aimed at assisting healthy people to function"

23. What is the expected outcome when working with a client who has experienced a crisis?
    a. Stabilization of mood with medications and return to previous levels of functioning
    b. Recovery from the crisis and return to precrisis level of functioning
    c. Recovery from the crisis with intense outclient therapy
    d. Recovery from the crisis with total adjustment at precrisis events

24. What statement below indicates that the nurse has an understanding of relaxation training?
    a. The nurse invites a client to the group and states that it is all right if he is "10 minutes late"
    b. A newly admitted client with a diagnosis of bipolar disorder comes to the group, and the nurse allows her to remain
    c. The nurse explains how anxiety relates to muscle tension and then establishes a quiet environment
    d. The nurse explains that there are differences in the relaxation experience and that "not everyone can use these techniques"

25. During a family session, a couple argues about religion and about what service to attend. The therapist recognizes this as
    a. Differentiation
    b. Family projection
    c. Triangling
    d. Emotional projection

26. A therapist is leading an inclient group. Which is most important to the development of the group process?
    a. Planning
    b. Goal setting
    c. Problem solving
    d. Reality orientation

27. During a family therapy session, two siblings blame their youngest sister for the family's problem. The target sibling is fulfilling the role of
    a. A hero
    b. A perfect child
    c. A defender
    d. A scapegoat

28. A client, age 21, comes to the emergency room with the complaint of inability to move the right arm. A complete medical examination reveals everything within normal limits. The most probable reason for the finding is
   a. Psychosomatic reaction
   b. Hysterical conversion
   c. Conversion reaction
   d. Anxiety reaction

29. A young man was found wandering around his town in a confused state. He is unable to state his name or where he is going. Which of the following describes his present state?
   a. Phobic reaction
   b. Bipolar disorder
   c. Hypochondriasis
   d. Dissociative disorder

30. In working with a client with antisocial personality disturbance, the nurse should adopt which attitude?
   a. Strict, punishing, restricting
   b. Accepting, supportive, indulgent
   c. Friendly, cautious, consistent
   d. Indulgent, pampering, concerned

31. Which would take the highest priority for the nurse caring for a client with bulimia?
   a. Communicate with a focus on feelings
   b. Assess for signs of anxiety
   c. Monitor meals to prevent purging
   d. Assess for signs of depression

32. A client is admitted with a diagnosis of long-term alcohol abuse. Which system is most seriously affected by alcohol abuse?
   a. Endocrine
   b. Cardiovascular
   c. Musculoskeletal
   d. Reproductive

33. A newly admitted client has needle tracks on the arms. The nurse must assess the client for early findings of narcotic withdrawal, which include
   a. Miosis, drowsiness, slurred speech
   b. Rhinorrhea, yawning, diaphoresis with chills
   c. Agitation, weakness, irritability
   d. Panic, auditory and visual hallucinations

34. A client is admitted to a psychiatric unit after taking an overdose of barbiturates. The diagnosis is depression. The next morning, as the nurse approaches the client bed, the client states, "I am too sick to be helped." What is the appropriate response?
    a. "I wouldn't try to help you if I didn't feel you were worth saving"
    b. "I know you can get well if you try"
    c. "You sound so hopeless. Will you share your thoughts with me?"
    d. "You are preoccupied, and that makes things worse"

35. A mental health client suffering from schizophrenia has been hearing voices telling him that he is "no good." The nurse notices the client becoming more agitated. The client tells the nurse that the voices are now telling him to "jump off the bridge." What is the nurse's priority intervention?
    a. Involve the client in groups so that his time is occupied
    b. Notify the physician and implement suicidal precautions
    c. Explain to the client that he is a worthwhile person
    d. Spend time with the client to encourage verbalization

36. A client diagnosed with bipolar disorder, manic phase, is prescribed lithium carbonate. The action of this medication is to
    a. Decrease depression
    b. Increase libido
    c. Increase affect
    d. Stabilize affect

37. The ways in which a schizophrenic client reduces anxiety includes
    a. Stuporous states alternating with excitement
    b. Loose associations and rationalization
    c. Ideas of reference and confabulation
    d. Withdrawal from reality and inappropriate laughter

38. A client tearfully insists that there are voices telling him that he is worthless. The nurse can help by saying the following
    a. "I understand you hear this so-called voice. I don't hear it"
    b. "I believe you are hearing this voice, but it is imaginary"
    c. "The voices you hear are probably other clients talking in the dayroom"
    d. "I don't hear the voice. Have you heard this voice in the past?"

39. A client who is paranoid schizophrenic should be involved in which activity?
    a. A nature walk
    b. A card game

    c.   Paint by numbers

    d.   A basketball game

40. When assessing a child with suspected autistic disorder, the nurse should look for

    a.   Failure to thrive

    b.   Attention deficits

    c.   No developed interpersonal skills

    d.   History of destructive behavior

41. Which is most commonly associated with dementia?

    a.   Ataxic gait and stance

    b.   Impaired memory and judgment

    c.   Delusions and confusion

    d.   Affective disturbances and memory impairment

42. A client experiences short-term memory loss. Which is an example of this?

    a.   Cannot remember what happened 3 weeks ago

    b.   Cannot remember the current president

    c.   Cannot remember three objects after 5 minutes

    d.   Cannot remember an anniversary

43. Which may be least effective to lessen the confusion in older adults?

    a.   Provide a night light in the bedroom and bathroom

    b.   Provide personal belongings such as pictures

    c.   Provide a structured schedule

    d.   For only the nurse to provide reality orientation

44. Delirium can be identified primarily and consistently by which characteristic?

    a.   Low IQ

    b.   Clouding of consciousness

    c.   Delusional thinking

    d.   Bizarre behavior

45. A client with Alzheimer's disease walks down the hall and calls the nurse by his wife's name. What should the response be?

    a.   "Hello, how are you?" This gives him a sense of being recognized.

    b.   "I'm not your wife." This points out reality.

    c.   "I am a nurse and you are in the hospital." This helps to orient him.

    d.   "You are always forgetting my name"

46. The ego usually copes with anxiety by rational means. If anxiety is painful, the individual copes by using a defense mechanism. Which statement is not true of defense mechanisms?
    a. They may operate consciously
    b. They may operate unconsciously
    c. They are considered maladaptive
    d. They may decrease or eliminate anxiety

47. During a conversion disorder, the client experiences paralysis. This symptom serves which function?
    a. Relieves anxiety and compromises the conflict
    b. Gets attention of others
    c. Allays anxiety and resolves the conflict
    d. Removes the conflict

ANSWERS, RATIONALES, AND TEST-TAKING TIPS

Rationales	Test-Taking Tips

1. Correct answer: d

The responsibility in a social relationship is shared between two individuals, where either individual may gain from the relationship. The responsibility in a therapeutic relationship is for the benefit of the client only. The other options also define the difference between social and therapeutic relationships, but they are not the primary difference.

The key word in the stem is "primary." This type of question indicates that all four options are correct and that you need to prioritize them. Generally the "responsibility" in any given situation would take priority over emotions, satisfaction, or information.

2. Correct answer: b

In regression the client resorts to behaviors of earlier developmental stages when a situation cannot get resolved through usual behaviors. Rationalization is an attempt to prove one's feelings are justifiable and acceptable to self and others. Repression is the unconscious or involuntary forgetting of painful events and conflicts. Suppression, although often listed as a defense mechanism, is really a conscious counterpart of repression; it is an intentional exclusion of material from consciousness.

Key clues in the stem are "returns to . . . a person much younger." Associate this backward behavior to an earlier time with regressing.

3. **Correct answer: a**

Suppression is the voluntary exclusion of anxiety-producing feelings, ideas, and situations. Sublimation is the acceptance of a socially approved substitute goal for a drive whose normal channel of expression is blocked. Example: a person who is impulsive and aggressive makes the football team as a star tackle). Substitution is an alternative gratification comparable to the one that would have been enjoyed if it were available. Example: a wife perceives her husband as cold and uncaring; she becomes a compulsive eater to experience good feelings, which substitute for the good feelings she felt when she dated her husband. Symbolization is the process of substituting an idea or object for repressed thoughts, feelings, or impulses; often these appear in dreams or fantasies.

Recall tips:
sup*press*ion = a pressed or scant emotion;
*"sub"*lim*a*tion = *"sub"*stitute society *a*pproved *a*ctivity—*a* in sublimation is a clue to approved activity;
substitution = substitute a gratification for emotions;
symbolization = sleep with symbols such as dreams or fantasies

4. **Correct answer: c**

Suppression is the voluntary exclusion of anxiety-producing feelings, ideas, and situations. Regression is a retreat in the face of stress to behavior characteristic of an earlier level of development. Denial is the unconscious refusal to admit to unacceptable behaviors

Recall that suppression is voluntary. Also note the clues in the words, "consciously not think about."

or ideas. Repression is the unconscious or involuntary forgetting of painful events and conflicts.

5. Correct answer: b

Sublimation is when the individual channels instinctual drives into socially or creatively acceptable activities. The other defense mechanisms are less compatible with mental health.

The key words in the stem are "fully compatible with mental health." In other words, which option would have or demonstrate a more positive direction?

6. Correct answer: c

Team meetings include all disciplines: medicine, nursing, social work, and occupational/recreational therapy. The client's case is reviewed, and treatment goals are revised.

If you have no idea of the correct answer, first note that the question is specific about a client's behaviors. Then cluster options *a, b,* and *d* under the category of meetings with a general or global focus. Select option *c,* which may most likely reflect an individual focus.

7. Correct answer: c

Clients admitted on an involuntary status have no right of refusal to treatment; when the status changes to voluntary, clients may then have the right to refuse treatment at that time unless they are posing a threat to themselves or others. The other actions in the options are included under the rights of clients; however, in a psychiatric setting these may be limited if deemed by the physician to be in the best interest of the involuntarily admitted client.

Involuntary admission or commitment may be of an emergency nature, 3 to 30 days; a temporary nature, 2 to 6 months; or an indefinite nature, subject to yearly review. Each state has criteria to defend in treating an involuntarily placed client in the event of the client's refusal.

8. **Correct answer: d**

   The examples in *a, b,* and *c* offer a reason to know about the client and his diagnosis. An employer may only obtain information directly from the client or if the client has signed a written consent to release this information to an employer.

   Confidentiality involves the disclosure of certain information to another person, and this is limited to authorized persons. Options *a, b,* and *c* are authorized persons to receive information.

9. **Correct answer: b**

   This statement encourages further conversation and asks for the client's perception before he accuses another client. Options *c* and *d* are judgmental statements. Option *a* is incomplete.

   Use the nursing process as a guide to select response *b.* Further assessment is done before interventions.

10. **Correct answer: c**

    In the orientation or introductory phase, trust and rapport must be established to move on to the working phase. Options *b* and *d* would be in the working phase. Option *a* is one small part of the orientation.

    Eliminate options *a, b,* and *d.* They are too narrow of responses for the question, which is asking for a more global or general focus.

11. **Correct answer: d**

    This is an attempt to present reality to the client. This also gives the client an opportunity to focus on the nurse's voice, which is the real voice. Restating is repeating to the client the main thought that the client expressed; no information is given in the

    The clue to the correct selection of option *d* is to note that the nurse's statement aligns with the word "reality" in option *d.*

stem about what the client
said. Clarification is asking
clients what they mean.
Focusing is the use
of questions or statements,
that help clients expand on
a thought.

12. **Correct answer: c**

This statement by the nurse
identifies feelings and gives
the client permission to
verbalize feelings about the
surgery. Options *a* and *b* offer
false reassurance. Option *d*
changes the subject from the
client to the physician.

The best response usually focuses
on the client. This guideline can
be applied to this question and
response.

13. **Correct answer: b**

ECT therapy results in a tonic-
clonic seizure, traditionally
called a grand mal seizure.
It involves the general brain,
the entire cerebral cortex,
and the diencephalon, which
includes the thalamus and
the hypothalamus. A partial
or focal seizure is in one
area of the brain. Most
ECT therapy is where only
one convulsion is produced.
If several convulsions are
induced immediately
following each other,
it is called multiple ECT.
A generalized seizure is
too general of an answer,
since the category of
general seizure includes
absence or petit mal
and tonic-clonic seizure
activity.

If you have no idea of the correct
answer, *go with what you know* to
be the most common seizure
activity—the client has tensed
(tonic) muscles, then goes into
jerking movements (clonic).

14. Correct answer: b

Chlorpromazine (Thorazine) is a major tranquilizer used to treat schizophrenia and to alleviate or decrease delusion and hallucination associated with the illness. Buspar, even though it is included in the sedative-hypnotic classification, is an antianxiety agent that does not produce sedation, euphoria, muscle relaxation, or physical dependence. It seems to have no potential for causing tolerance, no significant interaction with other sedative-hypnotics or alcohol, and no withdrawal syndrome. Buspar, given daily, has a lag period of about a week before effects begin; this is unlike the other sedative-hypnotics, which have a more immediate effect. Lithium, a mood stabilizer, is given for bipolar disorder. Prozac, an atypical antidepressant, has a lag period of 1 to 4 weeks before effects begin, as do the other antidepressants.

The best approach is to eliminate the drugs you can associate with types of problems. Most commonly, nurses are familiar with lithium and Prozac. Between the remaining choices, select Thorazine, since you know it has a calming effect and the client with schizophrenia may be more likely agitated and active.

15. Correct answer: d

Tardive dyskinesia, abnormal muscle movements primarily of the tongue, are first manifested by lip smacking and vermiform movements

Identify the associated part of the word in dyskinesia—kine—which pertains to movement. The only option with movement is *d*.

of the tongue. Cogwheel rigidity of the elbow is classic in Parkinson's. Dry mucous membranes usually result after anticholinergics are given. Akathisia is an inability to sit still.

16. **Correct answer: d**

This level is beyond the safe therapeutic range of 1.5 mEq/L. A level of 2.0 mEq/L is near the toxic range of this medication. A value of > 2.5 mEq/L is lethal. Normal therapeutic serum levels range from 0.5 to 1.5 mEq/L.

Eliminate option *c,* since a slightly elevated serum lithium level needs attention. If drug levels are below therapeutic range, the physician may not be routinely called; in such a case physicians will see the level the following day during client rounds. If you have no idea of the correct answer, select the abnormal option, *d,* rather than *a.*

17. **Correct answer: c**

The response by clients to antidepressants is usually delayed, with full effects of the medications taking 14 to 21 days.

Delete option *a,* since it is a nontherapeutic response giving reassurance—"not to worry." Eliminate option *b,* since it is too general of a response for this question. Eliminate option *d,* since it does not answer the concerns of the family member.

18. **Correct answer: c**

Prolixin deconate is a long-acting form administered IM. Because it is stored in the body fat, the effects can last up to 6 weeks. The other drugs have no long-acting forms.

The best approach, if you have no idea of the correct answer, is to make your best educated guess, take a deep breath, and go on to the next question, resist a reaction of emotional upset, which could carry over to the remaining questions. Recall tip: *Proli*xin can be given in a form that *prol*ongs its action.

19. Correct answer: b

Anafranil, a trycyclic antidepressant (TCA), is used in the treatment of obsessive-compulsive disorders if that is the primary diagnosis. Side effects are the same as for the other TCAs, except that there has been an 18% weight gain reported with Anafranil.

Remember to read slowly and carefully to note that the question is asking about the primary diagnosis. For this type of difficult question, make your best educated guess, take a deep breath, and go on the next question. Resist a reaction of emotional upset, which could carry over to the remaining questions. So what if you have two drug questions together? Tell yourself, "I'm doing well. Keep going!"

20. Correct answer: d

Antianxiety agents are usually prescribed for periods of stress and not as lifetime medications. If they have taken the antianxiety drug for longer than 4 months, clients are at risk for withdrawal symptoms if physical dependence has been established. The medication is taken as prescribed at home. Typically PRN doses are administered in institutions. The drugs may be titrated if clients are being weaned off the medication.

If you have no idea of the correct answer, *go with what you know—* antianxiety agents are used in time of stress, so select option *d.* Do not select the other options unless you are sure of the time, differences, or dosages.

21. Correct answer: a

The order of gr 1/150 is equal to 0.4 mg.

Associate that 60 min = 1 hr, with 60 mg = 1 gr. Therefore 1/150 gr = 0.4 mg.

22. Correct answer: b

Group therapy, with the use of structured groups, enables treatment of more individuals

Eliminate option *a,* since it is too general of a response to best answer the question about

in less time. Because members have similar problems, it provides a forum, through discussion by group members, to share coping methods, thus creating a greater awareness. In option *c* any group may have a period where group process becomes a focus in order to work through issues of the group members.

structured group. Eliminate option *c* with your knowledge of the four stages of group development: in stage 2, the initial stage, attention to group process is part of the focus to move along to the next stage, the working stage. Eliminate option *d* due to the extreme word, "intense," and because the group members are described as "healthy people." This is not enough information. Is it physical or mental health?

23. Correct answer: b

During a crisis the usual methods of coping become ineffective. All crisis events are self-limiting, which means they will have an end. Therapy includes working through the crisis with the client and establishing previous coping methods, or creating new and healthier coping methods and returning the individual to his/her precrisis level of functioning.

Eliminate option *a,* since the key words, "stabilization of the mood," are not even related to the question. Eliminate option *c* because of the too-restrictive "intense outclient therapy"; inclient therapy might be needed. Eliminate option *d* due to the words "*total* adjustment at precrisis events," which is an unrealistic outcome.

24. Correct answer: c

Relaxation training is used to teach clients to perform breathing and relaxation exercises while concentrating on a pleasant situation. This technique can help clients relax taut muscles, which in turn will help decrease anxiety. To perform relaxation techniques, the clients need to be able to concentrate and be still.

Eliminate option *a,* since being late would be disruptive to the group. Eliminate option *b,* since a newly diagnosed client with bipolar disorder would not be able to concentrate or be still in the manic or depressive state. Eliminate option *d* because the second part of the answer suggests a negative approach to learning. The first part of option *d* is a correct statement.

25. Correct answer: c

This is an emotional response when there is a problem in a relationship. Triangling represents dysfunctional efforts to reduce conflict. Triangling can be three people or two people and an object, group, or issue. Family projection is the process through which differentiation problems of parents are transmitted to one or more children, with the child becoming the scapegoat. Differentiation is the maintenance of intact boundaries, which enable people to freely move toward and away from each other.

Count the number of people, two, and add the issue, which makes three or a triangle in the discussion.

26. Correct answer: b

Goal setting is the main priority of inclient groups. Due to the short time clients are hospitalized, goals must be established, with the entire group working to achieve these goals. Planning is too global of a response to be the best answer. Problem solving is too narrow of a focus, also, note that not all groups need to problem solve. Reality orientation has nothing to do with the question.

The best approach is to eliminate the incorrect answers to arrive at the correct answer. A true-false approach could be used with each option to narrow them to either *a* or *b*. Reread the question and note that the question is asking about "the development of group process." Goal setting provides more direction than planning, so select option *b*.

27. Correct answer: d

Scapegoating is the projection of blame, anger, or suspicion onto another individual to avoid self-confrontation of an issue or situation.

Use your common sense to eliminate responses *a, b,* and *c* and choose *d*.

28. Correct answer: c

Conversion disorder, a type of somatoform disorder, is the finding of physical symptoms without an underlying organic cause. The symptoms, in reducing the anxiety, usually give clues to the conflict. Often clients display little concern about the conversion symptom and its resulting disability; this is termed *la belle indifference.*

Eliminate options *a* and *b,* since these are not appropriate terms. Eliminate option *d,* since it is too general of a description.

29. Correct answer: d

Dissociative disorders are reactions in which emotional conflicts are repressed, resulting in a split or separation of the personality. The end result is an altered consciousness or a confusion in identity.

Eliminate options *a, b,* and *d* by a logical approach. Phobic is related to fear, yet there is no information in the stem to suggest fear. Bipolar is associated with manic and depressive phases, yet there is no information given to support this choice. Hypochondriasis is chronic physical complaints, of which no information is given for this problem.

30. Correct answer: c

These individuals use manipulation as a defense mechanism. The nurse must convey a friendly attitude while maintaining caution to avoid the manipulative behavior. Consistency in treatment is helpful in reducing manipulative behavior.

The words in the other options that are wrong are as follows: strict, punishing, indulgent (permissive), and pampering. The other actions—restricting, accepting, supportive, and concerned—may be used in different degrees and within specific guidelines.

31. Correct answer: c

After meals the client is at high risk for acting out behaviors to reduce anxiety. Since purging will affect the client's physical status, the need for safety and for preservation of physiological integrity takes priority. Think of Maslow's hierarchy of needs.

If you have no idea of the correct answer, cluster options *a, b,* and *c* under the theme of feelings and mood, psychological focus. The only physiological focus is option *c.*

32. Correct answer: b

Excessive use of alcohol weakens the heart muscle and also causes small blood vessels to break, particularly in the cheeks, nose, and eyes, which are called spider angiomas. Alcohol eventually affects all body functions.

The key words in the stem are "most severely affected." If you have no idea of the correct answer, use the ABCs approach. There is no pulmonary to select, so select cardiovascular problems.

33. Correct answer: b

The early signs of narcotic withdrawal resemble symptoms of a flulike illness without the elevated temperature. Option *a* findings are the effects of narcotics. Option *c* presents findings of withdrawal that might occur 12 to 72 hours after withdrawal begins. Option *d* findings are associated with hallucinogenic drug usage.

Read the question carefully to note that it asks for the earliest findings of withdrawal. More commonly, early signs are more subtle, so the best approach is to select the group of findings that is the least severe. This is option *b.*

34. Correct answer: c

The client is verbalizing feelings of hopelessness. The nurse is requesting that the

If you have no idea of the correct answer, select the response that gets the client to talk. This is option *c.*

client share perceptions he/she feels at this time. The other options are incorrect, and they are barriers to therapeutic communication, since they reflect giving advice and making judgmental comments.

35. **Correct answer: b**

Often the schizophrenic client will respond to what the voices are telling him/her to do. It is imperative that the nurse initiate suicide precautions and notify the physician.

The clues in the stem are that the client becomes "agitated" and that the voices are "telling him to jump." These indicate a high-risk situation and guide the nurse to prioritize the client's safety.

36. **Correct answer: d**

Lithium carbonate is the drug of choice for bipolar disorder because it stabilizes the client's affect and returns him/her to a normal level of functioning without being excessively overactive or underactive in thought or actions.

Associate that bipolar means to have two extremes of behaviors and moods. Therefore the best answer is to stabilize and not to increase or decrease. Affect is defined as a feeling, mood, or emotional tone.

37. **Correct answer: d**

These individuals have flat or grossly inappropriate affects. They use withdrawn behavior and laughter as coping mechanisms to control their level of anxiety. Option *a* is more characteristic of the bipolar disorder due to the manic and depressive states. Schizophrenics use loose associations but do not rely

Schizophrenia is a group of mental disorders characterized by psychotic features, an inability to trust others, disordered thought process, and disrupted interpersonal relationships. The answer with the most psychotic flavor is *d*.

on rationalization as an anxiety reducer. Ideas of reference are incorrect interpretations of casual incidents and external events as having direct personal references. This might be found in the client having grandiose delusions. Confabulation is the making up of information for periods of time when the client cannot remember what happened.

38. **Correct answer: d**

The nurse, in this response, is presenting reality orientation to the client while trying to further assess whether this auditory hallucination is new or something the client experienced in the past. In options *a* and *b* the terms "so-called voice" and "it is imaginary" invalidate and belittle the client, who has already verbalized concern of worthlessness. The statement in option *c* ignores the concerns of the client.

If you have no idea of the correct answer, selecting the response that provides for further assessment will lead to the correct selection of *d*.

39. **Correct answer: c**

Noncompetitive, solitary activities requiring little concentration are best. Activities requiring minimal concentration may help to minimize hallucinations and delusions. Activities without other people may diminish the stimulation of suspiciousness and fearfulness.

If you have no idea of the correct answer, cluster the activities in options *a, b,* and *d* as those done with others. Select option *c,* a solitary activity.

40. Correct answer: c

The diagnosis of autism refers to aloneness, and the major finding is impairment of social interaction. Option *a* is not a finding in autism. Option *b* is incorrect; autistic children have short attention spans with impulsivity. Option *d* is too general; specifically, autistic self-injurious behaviors include head banging.

Recall tip: autism, think of being alone, with impaired interpersonal or communication skills.

41. Correct answer: b

The individual is unable to learn new information or to remember events or things well known in the past. The individual's judgment is also affected, which renders him/her unable to plan or cope with family, social, or financial issues. This represents the demented client's loss of intellectual ability. The other findings are not most commonly found in dementia.

For dementia recall that the mind deteriorates most commonly, and that this deterioration relates to normal functions of memory and judgment.

42. Correct answer: c

Short-term memory loss is when immediate recall and recent memory are seriously affected. The client may have difficult recalling what he/she had for lunch immediately after eating. Remote memory may be intact, although its deterioration usually indicates that a disease has progressed.

Short-term memory is the ability to recall events in the recent past. Two divisions of short-term memory are immediate memory (recall of information or data to which a person was just exposed) and recent memory (recall of events, information, and people from the past week or so). Long-term memory, also referred to as secondary memory or rote memory, is the recall of events, information, or people from the distant past. Primary memory is the conscious control for memory.

43. Correct answer: d

Lighting at night is needed because confused individuals tend to be more confused during the night. Pictures and personal belongings are familiar, offer comfort, and tend to reorient the client. Structure and consistency in the daily routine help to decrease confusion and disorientation.

Read carefully to note that the focus of the question is "least effective" action. If you are tired, tense, or read very quickly, you may read the question incorrectly and select a response to the question about actions to *lessen* confusion instead of about the *least* effective action.

44. Correct answer: b

Although symptoms and behaviors vary from client to client, memory impairment and clouding of the consciousness are dominant findings. As the disease progresses, all new information is rapidly forgotten. The findings in options *a, c,* and *d* may be found in other mental disorders.

If you have no idea of the correct answer, select a change in the level of consciousness, option *b.*

45. Correct answer: c

Clients with Alzheimer's disease become easily confused and forgetful. This statement by the nurse provides clarification of the client's surroundings and provides reality orientation.

Use common sense to select the correct answer.

46. Correct answer: c

While some defense mechanisms are used in a maladaptive fashion, others such as denial are fully compatible with good mental health.

If you have no idea of the correct answer, cluster options *a, b,* and *d* as statements without polarity of good or bad. Select option *c,* since its negative connotation suggests that defense mechanisms are negative. Be careful to reread the question before your final selection, since you may miss the key words, "is not true."

47. Correct answer: a

The underlying physical symptoms have no medical basis, but they relieve anxiety and help the individual avoid any current conflicts.

Option *b* may be a secondary gain from the physical symptom. The initial part of option *c* is correct, but the symptom does not resolve the conflict. Option *d* is incorrect.

BIBLIOGRAPHY

American Association of Retired Persons: *Domestic mistreatment of the elderly,* Washington, DC, 1992, American Association of Retired Persons.

American Psychiatric Association: *Diagnostic and statistical manual of mental disorders,* ed 4, Washington, DC, 1994, American Psychiatric Association.

Fortinash K and Holoday-Worret P: *Psychiatric nursing care plans,* St Louis, 1991, Mosby.

Haber J, McMahon AJ, Price-Hoskins P, and Sideleau BF: *Comprehensive psychiatric nursing,* ed 4, St Louis, 1992, Mosby.

Laraia M and Stuart G: *Quick psychopharmacology reference,* St Louis, 1991, Mosby.

Mount Sinai/Victim Services Agency Elder Abuse Project: *Elder mistreatment guidelines for health care professionals: Detection, assessment, and intervention,* Mount Sinai, 1988, Victim Services Agency Elder Abuse Project.

Pasquali, E, Arnold H, and Debasio N: *Mental health nursing: A holistic approach,* ed 3, St Louis, 1989, Mosby.

Rawlings R, Williams S, and Beck C: *Mental health-psychiatric nursing: A holistic life-cycle approach,* ed 3, St Louis, 1993, Mosby.

Stuart G and Sundeen S: *Principles and practice of psychiatric nursing,* ed 4, St Louis, 1993, Mosby.

Stuart G and Sundeen S: *Principles and practice of psychiatric nursing,* ed 5, St Louis, 1995, Mosby.

Rollant P: *Acing Multiple-Choice Tests,* American Journal of Nursing 1994 Career Guide, 18-21, 36, American Journal of Nursing.

Taylor, CM: *Essentials of psychiatric nursing,* ed 14, St Louis, 1993, Mosby.

INDEX

Instructions for Disk Start-Up

DOS Version

System Requirements

A computer with at least 324K of RAM (Random Access Memory) available is needed for this program. This computer must be IBM PC or 100% compatible.

For these examples we assume that your A drive is your floppy drive, and your C drive is your hard drive. Please substitute the letter of your floppy drive for A if your floppy drive letter is different. Substitute the letter of your hard drive for C if your hard drive letter is different.

Start-up (floppy drive):

1. Turn your computer on
2. At the prompt, insert the disk into your A drive
3. Type A: and press <Enter>
4. Type MOSBY and press <Enter>
5. Follow the instructions on the screen

Start-up (hard disk):

1. Turn your computer on
2. At the prompt, insert the disk into your A drive
3. Type C: and press <Enter>
4. Type MD\MOSBY and press <Enter>
5. Type CD\MOSBY and press <Enter>
6. Type COPY A:*.* and press <Enter>

The software is now installed on your hard drive. Once the software is installed, start the software by following these directions:

1. Type CD\MOSBY and press <Enter>
2. Type MOSBY and press <Enter>
3. Follow the directions on the screen

MAC Version

System Requirements

Mac 68XXX or Power Mac with a total of at least 1 MB of RAM is needed for this program.

Start-up:

1. Create a new folder on your hard disk called MOSBY.
2. Insert the disk into your floppy drive and open it.
3. Drag all items from the disk to the new folder.

The software is now installed on your hard drive. Once the software is installed, start the software by following these directions:

1. Open the MOSBY folder.
2. Select the MOSBY program.
3. Follow the directions on the screen.

WRITE DOWN THE PASSWORD THAT YOU HAVE SELECTED.
YOUR DISK WILL BE BRANDED WITH THIS INITIAL ENTRY.